Management of Infertility for the MRCOG and Beyond

Second edition

Edited by Siladitya Bhattacharya and Mark Hamilton

Series Editor: Jenny Higham

ISBN 978–1–904752–26–8

Published by the **RCOG Press** at the
Royal College of Obstetricians and Gynaecologists
27 Sussex Place, Regent's Park
London NW1 4RG

Registered Charity No. 213280

RCOG Press Editor: Jane Moody
Index: Liza Furnival
Design & typesetting: Saxon Graphics Ltd, Derby
Printed by Latimer Trend & Co. Ltd, Estover Road, Plymouth PL6 7PL, UK

Contents

About the authors

Premila Ashok MRCOG, MD
Consultant Gynaecologist, Ward 42/43, Aberdeen Royal Infirmary, Foresterhill, Aberdeen AB25 2ZD

Siladitya Bhattacharya MD, FRCOG
Professor of Reproductive Medicine and Head of Department, Department of Obstetrics and Gynaecology, University of Aberdeen, Aberdeen Maternity Hospital, Foresterhill, Aberdeen AB25 2ZD

Rafet Gazvani MD, MRCOG
Consultant Gynaecologist and Subspecialist in Reproductive Medicine and Surgery, Liverpool Women's Hospital, Crown Street, Liverpool L8 7SS

Mark Hamilton MD, FRCOG
Consultant Obstetrician and Gynaecologist, Aberdeen Maternity Hospital and Honorary Senior Lecturer, University of Aberdeen, Aberdeen AB25 2ZD

Haitham Hamoda MRCOG, DFFP
Specialist Registrar in Obstetrics and Gynaecology, Department of Obstetrics and Gynaecology, Ealing Hospital, Uxbridge Road, Middlesex UB1 3HW

Susan Logan MRCOG, MD
Subspecialty Trainee in Sexual and Reproductive Health Care, Department of Obstetrics and Gynaecology, Aberdeen Maternity Hospital, Foresterhill, Aberdeen AB25 2ZD

Ashalatha Shetty MD, MRCOG, MRCP(II), DGO
Consultant Obstetrician and Fetal Maternal Subspecialist, Department of Obstetrics and Gynaecology, Aberdeen Maternity Hospital, Foresterhill, Aberdeen AB25 2ZD

Allan Templeton MD, FRCOG, FMed Sci, FRCP
Regius Professor, Department of Obstetrics and Gynaecology, University
of Aberdeen, Aberdeen Maternity Hospital, Foresterhill, Aberdeen
AB25 2ZD

Series Editor: Jenny M Higham MD FRCOG FFFP ILTM
Head of Undergraduate Medicine/Consultant Gynaecologist, Faculty of
Medicine, Imperial College London, South Kensington Campus,
Sir Alexander Fleming Building, London SW7 2AZ

Abbreviations

AMH	anti-müllerian hormone
BMI	body mass index
DBCP	dibromochloropropane
CBAVD	congenital bilateral absence of the vas deferens
cGMP	cyclic guanosine monophosphate
CFTR	cystic fibrosis transmembrane conductance regulator
CMV	cytomegalovirus
DHEA-S	dehydroepiandrosterone sulphate
ERPOC	evacuation of retained products of conception
FAI	free androgen index
FSH	follicle-stimulating hormone
GIFT	gamete intrafallopian transfer
GnRH	gonadotrophin-releasing hormone
GP	general practitioner
hCG	human chorionic gonadotrophin
HFEA	Human Fertilisation and Embryology Authority
hMG	human menopausal gonadotrophin
HRT	hormone replacement therapy
HSG	hysterosalpingogram
ICSI	intracytoplasmic sperm injection
IgA	immunoglobulin A
IgG	immunoglobulin G
IUI	intrauterine insemination
IVF	in vitro fertilisation
LH	luteinising hormone
LHRH	luteinising hormone-releasing hormone
M/ml	million per millilitre
NICE	National Institute for Health and Clinical Excellence
OHSS	ovarian hyperstimulation syndrome
PCOS	polycystic ovary syndrome
PID	pelvic inflammatory disease
RCT	randomised controlled trial

SHBG	sex hormone-binding globulin
TRH	thyroid-releasing hormone
TSH	thyroid-stimulating hormone
WHO	World Health Organization
ZIFT	zygote intrafallopian transfer

Preface

This concise volume – completely up to date and written by experts in their fields – is certain to be popular as the demands on the gynaecologist from patients seeking help with their suboptimal fertility continues to grow. Issues related to fertility never seem to be far from the gaze of the media and this, together with the Internet journeys of our patients, can sometimes make them appear the 'experts'. Therefore, as obstetricians and gynaecologists we need to ensure that we are up to date, informed and knowledgeable to successfully engage with our patients.

In each chapter of this revised edition, current evidence-based knowledge is concisely summarised and the contentious issues are addressed. This book will be of use not only for those updating their knowledge but also will be of great value to those who are hoping to impress their examiners.

This eagerly awaited volume is a succinct contemporary overview of infertility management. I hope you enjoy it.

Jenny Higham
December 2006

Foreword

The management of infertility in the 21st century needs to tread a careful line between the rapid pace of technological advances and the relative paucity of robust evaluative data supporting such developments. As in the previous edition, this book presents an overview of evidence-based fertility treatment and highlights areas where such evidence is lacking.

In this edition, all the chapters have been extensively revised to include new sources of evidence and reflect changes in practice. We hope that this book will continue to meet the needs of candidates for the MRCOG as well as specialists who wish to consult a concise, readily accessible text.

Siladitya Bhattacharya and Mark Hamilton
December 2006

1 Introduction

Introduction

Infertility affects one in seven couples in industrialised countries. There has been no major change in prevalence in recent years but more couples are seeking help than previously. This is associated with a greater awareness of the problem and also the availability of more effective treatment, particularly in vitro fertilisation (IVF). There are, however, wide variations in clinical practice, and dissatisfaction with services continues to be highlighted by patient groups.

Infertility can cause considerable psychological distress to couples. The United Nations states that reproductive health is 'a state of complete physical, mental and social wellbeing and not merely the absence of disease or infirmity in all matters relating to the reproductive system and to its function and processes'. Infertility should therefore be considered a disease worthy of investigation and treatment.

Definitions of infertility vary considerably, particularly in relation to the duration of regular unprotected intercourse (Box 1.1). Circumstances will differ but couples should be considered individually and seen whenever they think there is a problem. Often, there are factors such as the woman's age, previous surgery or irregular periods that warrant investigation earlier than the usual one or two years of trying. Generally, couples appreciate a service that provides rapid and efficient assessment, frank discussion of prognosis and a clearly agreed plan of management. Two major issues have shaped practice in recent years:

Box 1.1 Definition of infertility

Primary infertility Couples have never conceived at any stage

Secondary infertility Couples have had a pregnancy, although not necessarily a successful one

---

- the introduction of an evidence-based approach to management and, in particular, treatment
- the increasing availability of assisted reproduction.

One of the major problems in the current provision of services is insufficient access to IVF and related techniques.

Epidemiology

Despite differences in approach and definition, most studies indicate that approximately 15% of all couples will experience difficulties in conceiving (Box 1.2). Of these, about 50% will be subfertile rather than infertile and will eventually go on to conceive, either spontaneously or with the help of simple advice and remedies. The other 50% will remain infertile and will require more sophisticated treatment, of the kind usually only available in established infertility clinics. In all, approximately 50% of these will have primary infertility and the other 50% will have secondary infertility. Current information also suggests a higher incidence of miscarriage and ectopic pregnancy among subfertile women.

A number of studies now indicate that the likelihood of a spontaneous pregnancy occurring in a subfertile woman is greatly influenced by her age, the duration of infertility and the occurrence of a previous pregnancy. This is the case for all categories of infertility but especially for unexplained infertility, and this is further addressed in Chapter 7. These issues are clearly important for clinical management and also for assessing the outcome of new interventions and treatment. The woman's characteristics also have a major effect on the likelihood of any treatment being successful.

KEY POINTS
- Approximately 15% of all couples will experience difficulties in conceiving.
- A young woman with a short duration of infertility and a previous pregnancy is much more likely to become pregnant without treatment than an older woman with a longer duration of infertility and no pregnancies.

Box 1.2 Prevalence of infertility
- Couples who will experience infertility   15%
- Couples whose infertility remains unresolved   8%
- Those with primary infertility   4%
- Those with secondary infertility   4%

Aetiology

In this book, aetiology will be addressed in the context of the management of the individual clinical problems. Generally speaking causal factors can be associated with:

- lifestyle (e.g. weight and smoking)
- genetic causes (e.g. sex chromosome anomalies and Kallmann syndrome)
- acquired causes (e.g. following injury and infection).

LIFESTYLE

Smoking, both male and female, has been associated with subfertility as well as poorer treatment outcomes. Although the association is quite strong, particularly in women, a causal relationship has yet to be clearly established. It is important to determine, when taking the history, whether there are any other lifestyle factors that may be contributory. Increasingly, also, obesity is recognised as a major issue in the management of infertility.

GENETIC CAUSES

The clinical presentation will usually provoke appropriate investigations in relation to genetic causes but there are now additional concerns about the implications for the offspring. Using assisted reproduction techniques, the infertility of this generation can often be overcome but in the process the problem may be handed on to the next generation.

ACQUIRED CAUSES

In relation to acquired problems, two stand out in the female:

- the consequences of surgery on the reproductive tract
- infection of the upper tract, particularly when caused by *Chlamydia trachomatis.*

The association between chlamydia and tubal infertility is now well established. It is accepted that chlamydia is the major preventable cause of tubal disease in the Western world. It may turn out to be the major preventable cause of infertility when its effect on the male is also considered.

- Smoking has been associated with subfertility as well as poorer treatment outcomes.
- Obesity is now recognised as a major issue in infertility.
- Genetic problems may be overcome, but may be passed on to the next generation.
- Chlamydia may be the major preventable cause of infertility.

Diagnostic categories

Couples are usually managed in the context of the major diagnostic category to which they have been assigned. These categories are based not so much on diagnosis but on functional and pragmatic considerations that facilitate treatment (Table 1.1). However, not all couples will fit neatly into one category and several problems may have to be managed simultaneously, such as inducing ovulation in a woman who is anovulatory in order to carry out donor insemination.

The distribution of couples in each of the diagnostic categories will vary from clinic to clinic depending on referral patterns: typical figures are shown. Couples with primary infertility are more frequent in all of the categories except tubal, where secondary infertility is more frequent. This highlights the fact that pregnancy is a risk factor for the development of tubal disease, presumably associated with opportunities for ascending infection, whether after early or late pregnancy. Table 1.1 highlights the importance of investigating the male partner in cases of secondary infertility, even where he has been a partner in a recent pregnancy.

Table 1.1 Diagnostic categories and distribution of couples with primary and secondary infertility

Diagnostic category	Infertility	
	Primary (%)	Secondary (%)
Male	25	20
Ovulation	20	15
Tubal	15	40
Endometriosis	10	5
Unexplained	30	20

Prevention of infertility

Unfortunately the opportunities for the prevention of infertility appear to be limited. However, there is now much more awareness of the importance of appropriate surgical technique when operating on young women whose fertility may be an issue. Similarly, the prevention of chlamydial infection is receiving much more attention, although gynaecologists need to be much more aware of the risks of ascending infection in women. Highly sensitive nucleic acid-based tests have now been developed to detect chlamydia and these can be carried out in first-void urine samples or vulval swabs, as well as cervical swabs. Any woman at risk, and this particularly applies to women under the age of 25 years, who are having uterine instrumentation for any reason, should be tested for chlamydia.

Eventually reductions in the prevalence of chlamydia will result from better public awareness as well as population-based screening.

Advice about the consequences of postponing childbirth is also seen as increasingly important.

KEY POINT
- Any woman at risk who is having uterine instrumentation for any reason should be tested for the presence of *C. trachomatis*.

Effective treatments

In recent years a much more critical approach to the effective management of the infertile couple has emerged. Evaluation of the literature in a systematic way has demonstrated that many of the treatments previously used in the management of the infertile couple were ineffective and should no longer be used. Areas where the evidence does not support treatment include:

- drug treatment of the male
- drug treatment for infertility-related endometriosis
- (probably) the use of clomifene for unexplained infertility.

Where there is continuing uncertainty, a treatment should only be used within the context of randomised clinical trials.

At the same time, there has been increasing dependence on more complex treatments, including ovarian stimulation and intrauterine insemination and, particularly, IVF and related techniques. These techniques are not effective in all circumstances, having as they do a relatively low success rate for each cycle of intervention.

As previously noted, it is now well established that a number of patient characteristics have enormous importance in predicting the likelihood of a spontaneous pregnancy, whatever the clinical diagnosis. A young woman with a short duration of infertility and a previous pregnancy has a high likelihood of achieving a further spontaneous pregnancy (that is, without intervention or treatment) and it would be very difficult for any of the interventions at our disposal to match this likelihood. It may therefore be appropriate to postpone treatment in these circumstances in the expectation that a pregnancy will occur naturally. The strength of these factors has been quantified in a number of studies, and the results from one such study carried out in Canada are shown in Table 1.2.

These factors are also the main determinants in assessing the outcome of any intervention. Thus, a young woman in her twenties might expect a greater than 30% chance of a live birth following IVF whereas a woman in her early forties would expect a less than 10% chance.

COST EFFECTIVENESS

Assessing cost effectiveness is a much more difficult issue. Comparing two similar treatments, one using an expensive drug and the other using a cheap drug, may be easy, particularly if they both have similar pregnancy rates. However, the cheaper drug may be administered over several cycles and produce as good a pregnancy rate as the more expensive drug given for one cycle, but with fewer adverse effects and complications. The issue of cost effectiveness then becomes much more difficult; particularly where there is a risk of multiple pregnancy and associated perinatal morbidity. Nonetheless, the importance of assessing cost and benefits, particularly within the context of randomised studies,

---

KEY POINT
- The effectiveness of a treatment is greatly dependent on the woman's age, duration of infertility and previous pregnancy history.

Table 1.2   Patient characteristics and the likelihood of a live birth (data from Collins *et al.* 1995)

	Odds of live birth	95% confidence limits
Secondary infertility	1.8	1.2–2.7
< 3 years of infertility	1.7	1.1–2.5
Female < 30 years	1.5	1.1–2.2

is now acknowledged when assessing the overall effects of infertility management.

Unwanted effects of treatment

Three unwanted effects of treatment are highlighted. These are:

- the emotional consequences
- multiple births
- the cancer risk.

EMOTIONAL CONSEQUENCES

The inevitable emotional consequences of infertility can be diminished by a number of important measures. These include the adequate provision of information, efficient provision of services and more awareness among professionals of the psychological and emotional impact of infertility. Similarly, coordination of investigations between the different levels of service and more support when giving the results of tests, particularly if the news is not good, can all help to diminish the problem. The issues that cause most distress to patients are insensitive staff, poor coordination of services, inadequate standards of treatment, lack of information and lack of support when most needed (Box 1.3). Although there is no direct evidence that counselling improves the outcome of fertility treatment, there is good evidence that counselling reduces distress and there is some evidence that distress may adversely affect the outcome.

MULTIPLE BIRTHS

The high rate of multiple births resulting from infertility treatment remains a major concern. The medical, social and financial consequences are considerable, chiefly because of the excessive morbidity among the survivors of high-order multiple births (triplets or more) as well as the increased morbidity associated with the far more numerous

---

Box 1.3 Ranking of parents' views about infertility management (data from Souter *et al.* 1998)

- The information and explanation given (including written information)
- The doctor's attitude (listening and supportive)
- The way investigations are done (quickly and efficiently)
- Help with emotional side (counselling)
- Waiting time at clinic (and more frequent appointments)

---

twins. The problems arise mainly from ovulation induction and IVF treatment. In ovulation induction, multiple pregnancies are associated with the difficulties in monitoring follicular development. Previous guidance has recommended that:

- all centres should adopt protocols that minimise the risk of multiple pregnancy and ovarian hyperstimulation
- all patients undergoing ovulation induction should be given information about the risks of multiple pregnancy, ovarian hyperstimulation and the possibility of fetal reduction
- ovulation induction with gonadotrophins should only be performed in circumstances which permit daily monitoring of ovarian response (in practice, this means daily access to ultrasound monitoring)
- clinics should clearly define the criteria for abandoning cycles and should be prepared to abandon cycles where there is any risk of multiple follicular development.

With IVF, the problem relates to the number of embryos transferred in treatment cycles. Although there is now a limit in the UK of two embryos in any cycle, and there is increasing evidence that two embryos will suffice in most situations, this does not remove the risk of twins and the resultant increased morbidity and costs. It has to be recognised that clinicians and couples feel under considerable pressure to maximise pregnancy rates but there is an increasing view that multiple gestation, including twin pregnancy, is an unacceptable consequence of these pressures.

RISK OF CANCER

There has been increasing concern in recent years about a possible link between drugs given for infertility treatment and the subsequent risk of cancer, particularly ovarian cancer. It is well established that nulliparous women, and particularly infertile women, are at greater risk of developing ovarian cancer than parous women but the effects of treatment are less clear. Recent studies should reassure us that any additional effect of drug treatment, if present, is likely to be small and does not affect women who conceive with such treatment. Nevertheless, the association between ovarian cancer risk and gonadotrophins or prolonged clomifene use remains uncertain and all women should be counselled about the putative risks of ovarian cancer associated with ovarian induction therapy. There is also a responsibility on practitioners to limit the use of gonadotrophins to the lowest effective dose and duration of use.

Context of care

Much of the initial investigation and management of the infertile couple can be carried out within primary care. It is important, however, that there are agreed protocols, based on national guidelines, for investigation and referral. Inevitably, the resources and facilities available in secondary care will vary considerably and these will depend on the local circumstances and the population served. Whatever the situation, a basic minimum set of requirements is envisaged:

- The couple should always be managed as a couple.
- Their management should always be discussed in the context of their particular clinical situation and where necessary supported by appropriate written information.
- Patients should be fully involved in decisions regarding their treatment.
- Patients should have access to expert advice and counselling to help them in making their choices and in managing their infertility.
- Secondary care should take place in a dedicated infertility clinic in which there are appropriate facilities and access to trained staff, including doctors, nurses and counsellors.

Guidelines anticipate that these issues should be addressed by all of those involved in the provision of infertility care, including not just the practitioners, but also patients and the commissioning services. Access to tertiary care, particularly IVF, is still limited within the National Health Service in the UK but it is important that patients should have access to the highest available standards and quality of care, wherever they present. This remains a problem despite national guidelines recently issued.

Summary

The two aspects of care that are ranked most highly by patients are the information and explanation given and the doctor's attitude. Many patients also indicate that they would like more written information. Many feel that they are leaving clinics with unresolved questions and without a clear plan of future management. Similarly, prolonged investigation has been a frequent source of frustration and difficulty to many couples. The use of protocols that minimise unnecessary investigations and prevent duplication of tests should facilitate the process of management as well as referral to secondary and tertiary care.

Recommended reading

Collins JA, Burrows EA, Wilan AR. The prognosis for live birth among untreated infertile couples. *Fertil Steril* 1995;64:22–8.

National Collaborating Centre for Women's and Children's Health. *Fertility: Assessment and Treatment for People with Fertility Problems*. London: RCOG Press; 2004.

Souter VL, Penney G, Hopton JL, Templeton AA. Patient satisfaction with the management of infertility. *Hum Reprod* 1998;13:1831–6.

2 The initial assessment of the infertile couple

Introduction

Infertility is a major public health problem and it is essential that limited public resources are used prudently in its management. The importance of efficient mechanisms for referral and investigation of the infertile couple cannot therefore be overestimated. Region-wide protocols of basic investigation[1-3] are a valuable asset for those involved in the planning of services. Adherence to such protocols facilitates appropriate and timely investigation and minimises the risks of delay and repetition of tests which couples find particularly demoralising.

Pragmatic definition of infertility

In counselling couples experiencing difficulty in achieving pregnancy, account must be taken of what is a realistic expectation of fertility in normal circumstances. Epidemiological data indicate that conception occurs in 84% of women within 12 months of ceasing contraception and in 92% by 2 years.[4] Thus, many would suggest that infertility should be defined as failure to conceive after at least 2 years of unprotected intercourse. In actual fact, there may be particular pressures, which may lead to couples seeking advice before two years have elapsed.

PRIMARY CARE

The role of the general practitioner (GP) is crucial.[5] Infertility represents a deeply personal problem and many individuals will prefer to discuss intimate matters with someone they know and trust. The support that the GP can provide in terms of counselling and preliminary investigations is an excellent foundation for provision of care. Once referral is made to a specialist clinic, increasing demands on couples' time, the indignity of some of the investigations and the invasion of privacy that accompanies them, adds to the stresses imposed on couples. It is recognised that infertility investigation and treatment pose real threats to domestic stability and the GP, through knowledge of the couple and their families, may be in the best position to provide support for those at greatest risk.

All patients should be seen as couples in appropriate surroundings. Facilities should be available to permit examination of both partners and with sufficient time, usually half an hour, to make an adequate overall assessment of the problem.

HOSPITAL CARE

This should be provided in a setting under the clinical direction of a consultant gynaecologist with a special interest in infertility. Patients should be seen in a dedicated infertility clinic with appropriate appointment times to permit thorough evaluation. A team system should be established involving medical, nursing, laboratory (endocrinology and semenology) and counselling personnel to facilitate a consistent and coordinated approach. The level of treatment options available will depend on the expertise of, and the facilities available to, staff at each centre.

KEY POINTS
- Infertility is defined as failure to conceive after at least 2 years of unprotected intercourse.
- All patients should be seen as couples in appropriate surroundings.
- A team system should be established to facilitate a consistent and coordinated approach to care.

The infertility consultation

Any couple worried about their fertility should be seen by their GP, regardless of the duration of their infertility. It is unusual for couples to present if this is less than 1 year. In these circumstances, unless there is a clear indication on the basis of history or examination of either partner, further investigation is usually unnecessary. Merely providing the couple with an outline of their excellent potential fertility over the next year may be all that is required to set their minds at rest. However, couples that present early may themselves have particular concerns or be aware of a problem that merits sympathetic discussion. A little more urgency may be required in the investigation of couples where the female partner is over 35 years of age.

Steps in the process of investigation of infertility should be discussed at the outset with the couple, in the expectation that all necessary tests would be complete within 4 months. The sequence with which tests are performed is, to some extent, standardised for all but may vary if history or examination findings suggest otherwise. Initial investigations are inexpensive, non-invasive and likely to yield useful information.

Points requiring particular attention in the history and examination of the couple are shown in Tables 2.1 and 2.2. A psychological assessment of the impact of perceived infertility on individual and couple would also be required.

KEY POINTS

- The success rate for the treatment of infertility declines with increasing duration of infertility and increasing age.
- All necessary tests should be completed within 4 months; these are inexpensive, noninvasive and likely to yield useful information.
- A genital examination should be performed even without a positive finding in the history. A small proportion of men will exhibit unsuspected genital pathology, which may have an important bearing on their health in general, and not just their infertility.
- Adnexal pathology such as endometriosis should be borne in mind, particularly for those with a suggestive history.

Appropriate initial investigations

MALE

Semen analysis remains the most important facet of male investigation. In most instances a single analysis, if normal, will suffice. If an abnormality is found then the sample should be repeated, usually after 1 month. In order to avoid unhelpful and frustrating duplication, it is desirable for GP-referred assessments to take place in the same laboratory that serves the clinic to which the couple may ultimately be referred. It is imperative that clear instructions regarding the period of abstinence and method of production and transport of specimens are provided by the laboratory. The production of two specimens minimises the chance of laboratory error and the likelihood that a transient illness such as influenza might provide a misleading indication of abnormal spermatogenesis. What constitutes a normal result is perhaps a matter for debate. Large laboratories may have their own local population-based normal ranges but, in the absence of such information, the World Health Organization values for definition of normality can be applied (Box 2.1).

Table 2.1   Investigation of infertility: history

Area of investigation	History — Male	History — Female
Infertility	Previous evidence of fertility and, if so, with present partner or not Duration of infertility and time to achieve previous pregnancies, if any	Duration of infertility Length and type of previous contraceptive use Fertility in previous relationships as well as present liaison Previous investigation and treatment Fertility subsequently, if known, of any former partners Previous investigations and treatment for infertility

Medical	Sexually transmitted disease
	
	Epididymitis
	
	Mumps orchitis
	Testicular maldescent
	Chronic disease
	Drug/alcohol abuse
	Recent febrile illness
	Recurrent urinary tract infection
		Menstrual:
		  Cyclicity
		  Pain
		  Bouts of amenorrhoea
		  Menorrhagia
		  Intermenstrual bleeding
		Number of previous pregnancies, including abortions and ectopic pregnancies
		Any associated sepsis
		Time to initiate previous pregnancies

Surgical	Hemiorrhaphy Testicular injury Torsion Orchidopexy Vasectomy	Especially abdominal or pelvic surgery
Occupational	Exposure to toxic substances including chemicals, radiation Time away from home through work	

Sexual	Onset of puberty:
	  Coital habits
	  Premature ejaculation
	  Libido
	  Impotence
	Use and knowledge of the fertile period
		Coital frequency/timing, including knowledge of the fertile period

Table 2.2   Investigation of infertility: examination

Area of investigation	Examination
Male	
General	Height, weight, BMI, blood pressure
	Fat and hair distribution
	Evidence of hypoandrogenism and gynaecomastia
Groin	Exclude inguinal hernia (patient in upright position)
	Check for inguinal mass, e.g. ectopic testicle
Genitalia	Note site of testicles in scrotum
	Palpate testes and note testicular volume, using an orchidometer
	Palpate epididymes for modularity or tenderness
	Check presence and normality of vasa deferentia
	Check for presence of a varicocoele
	Examine penis for any structural abnormality, e.g. hypospadias
Female	
General	Height, weight, BMI, blood pressure
	Fat and hair distribution (Ferriman Galwey score to quantify hirsutism)
	Note presence or absence of acne and galactorrhoea
Abdomen	Check for abdominal masses or tenderness
Pelvis	Assess state of the hymen
	Assess normality of clitoris and labia
	Assess vagina, looking for such problems as infection or vaginal septa
	Check for presence of cervical polyps
	Assess accessibility of the cervix for insemination
	Record uterine size, position, mobility and tenderness
	Perform cervical smear (if appropriate)

Additional investigations may be required if the semen analysis fails to meet these criteria.

FEMALE

At the outset it is advisable to ensure that the woman is rubella immune and that she is taking folic acid (0.4 mg/day) to reduce the chance of neural tube defects. A higher dose (5 mg/day) should be prescribed if there is a past history of neural tube defect or if the patient is on anti-epileptic medication.

The next step centres on the need to demonstrate that the woman is ovulating. This is almost certainly the case if she has a regular monthly cycle. Laboratory evidence may be obtained through measurement of serum progesterone in the putative luteal phase of the menstrual cycle. Levels should be in excess of 30 nmol/l 7 days after ovulation (depending on local laboratory levels). For this reason, sampling should be arranged for day 21 in a 28-day cycle, with serial checks made beyond this point if the cycle is more prolonged. Results should be interpreted only in relation to the onset of the subsequent period. If the level is below 30 nmol/l, the test should be repeated in a subsequent cycle. In the absence of any clues in history or examination to suggest the possibility of an endocrine disorder, these tests would be sufficient. If there is a history of irregular menstruation or periods of amenorrhoea, especially if associated with galactorrhoea, hirsutism or obesity, additional biochemical tests are appropriate. These would include measurement of follicle-stimulating hormone (FSH), luteinising hormone (LH), thyroid-stimulating hormone (TSH) and prolactin, timing sampling for the early follicular phase if the women were having periods. If significant hirsutism is present, testosterone, sex hormone-binding globulin (SHBG) and adrenal androgens should be measured. There is no evidence that the use of temperature charts and LH detection methods to time intercourse improves outcome and their use should be discouraged.

The investigations outlined above can be initiated by the GP but they also provide the basis for hospital investigation. It is useful to send the couple a questionnaire to supplement the information provided in the GP's referral letter.

Valuable time can then be saved if routine questions in respect of history and previous investigations can be avoided in the clinic.

General advice for practitioners to give to patients

Table 2.3 gives a summary of general advice. There is reasonable evidence to support the suggestion that smoking reduces female fertility, while it is known that smoking may affect sperm quality. In men, there is evidence that high alcohol intake can compromise reproductive function, as well as general health. There is less convincing evidence linking alcohol and female fertility but intake in excess of two units/day of alcohol is thought to be detrimental to the fetus in pregnancy. Women with a body mass index (BMI) in excess of 30 should be encouraged to lose weight. This may cause a resumption in ovulation in women who are anovulatory or, alternatively, may enhance the response to treatment where instituted. Women with a BMI below 19 with irregular periods or amenorrhoea should be advised that increasing their body weight will increase their chances of conception. Hyperthermia is likely to adversely affect sperm quality (see also Chapter 3).

Further tests

FEMALE

Where preliminary investigations suggest that the woman is ovulating and sperm production is satisfactory, pelvic assessment should be undertaken (Table 2.4). In women who do not have an identified risk factor (past history of pelvic inflammatory disease, previous ectopic pregnancy, symptoms or examination findings suggestive of endometriosis) then the hysterosalpingogram (HSG) is a suitable first-line investigation. With the above comorbidities, laparoscopy and dye hydrotubation is the investigation of choice unless the patient is unsuitable for surgery, in order to identify those cases with endometriosis and peritubal adhesions. HSG may be helpful in those cases where pelvic pathology has been found at laparoscopy and further information is required to clarify the extent of tubal disease and perhaps the suitability of such patients for tubal surgery.

Table 2.3 Summary of general advice given to patients

Advice	Action
Smoking	Advise both partners to stop
Alcohol	Both partners to limit alcohol intake if attempting to conceive
Body mass index (BMI)	Encourage women with a BMI in excess of 30 to lose weight
Temperature	Advise men to wear loose fitting underwear and trousers and avoid conditions that might elevate scrotal temperature

Table 2.4 Summary of pelvic investigations

Procedure	Comments
Hysterosalpingogram (HSG)	First-line investigation if pelvic pathology unlikely Reliable test for ruling out tubal occlusion
Laparoscopy + dye hydrotubation	Investigation of choice if pelvic pathology suspected Identifies endometriosis and peritubal adhesions
Hysterosalpingo-contrast-ultrasonography	Used to visualise intrauterine and tubal pathology Potential alternative to HSG Yet to gain widespread popularity
Hysteroscopy	Prospective studies awaited May be feasible in women with identified intrauterine abnormalities
Screening for chlamydia	Recommended for women considered at risk Antibiotic prophylaxis may be an alternative Collaboration with a genitourinary clinic advisable

Present evidence would suggest that minor abnormalities of the uterine cavity such as tubocornual polyps are of little importance in the genesis of infertility. The use of ultrasound in combination with sono-reflective contrast media to visualise intrauterine and tubal pathology has been promoted as an alternative outpatient investigation but has yet to gain widespread popularity. Prospective studies are also awaited to determine whether hysteroscopy may have a part to play in the routine investigation of infertile women although in women with identified intrauterine abnormalities, hysteroscopic surgery may be feasible. Before any uterine instrumentation, women considered at risk (generally those less than 30 years of age) should be screened for *C. trachomatis* using an appropriately sensitive technique. Alternatively, antibiotic prophylaxis, for example with doxycycline or azithromycin, may be considered. It is recommended that where chlamydial infection is discovered there should be a local mechanism whereby the disease can be notified and sexual partners treated. Collaboration with a genitourinary clinic is advisable.

MALE

The capacity of sperm to fertilise an egg depends on a complex series of biological events including transport to the site of fertilisation, sperm-egg recognition, the acrosome reaction and fusion of the sperm to the oocyte. It has been claimed that the postcoital test is useful in providing information about sperm function in the male.[6] However, systematic review of the literature would suggest that the test lacks validity for routine use. Nevertheless, if sexual dysfunction is suspected, or the male partner cannot or will not provide a semen sample for analysis, the postcoital test may have a place, even at an early stage in investigations. It is crucial that the test is done at the correct stage in the cycle; that is, at the time of maximal cervical mucus production prior to ovulation. Inappropriate timing of the test may provide misleading information and cause unnecessary concern. Ideally, mucus production should be assessed daily using an objective method. Occasionally, mucus production may be poor until the day of the beginning of the LH surge and this may indicate a functional problem within the cervix, an unusual situation even in cases where there has been previous cervical surgery. This need for precise timing leads to a sex-on-demand approach to investigation, which may produce additional strain and tension for an already overburdened couple trying to cope with the stress of their infertility and their associated loss of self-esteem.

Other tests of sperm function including computerised analysis of sperm movement characteristics and sperm cervical mucus penetration tests, among others, are not recommended for routine use, nor is the testing for antisperm antibodies in semen. The place for such tests will be discussed in Chapter 3.

KEY POINTS

- Where preliminary investigations have suggested that the woman is ovulating and sperm production is satisfactory, pelvic assessment should be undertaken.
- HSG is suitable for pelvic assessment if pelvic pathology is unlikely.
- Laparoscopy and dye hydrotubation is the investigation of choice if pelvic pathology is suspected.
- If sexual dysfunction is suspected or the male partner cannot or will not provide a semen sample for analysis, the postcoital test may have a place at an early stage in investigations.

Summary

The preliminary assessment of egg and sperm availability, together with a determination that the gametes can meet, should provide a diagnosis for the majority of couples. In most cases, a prognosis, usually favourable, can also be provided. Appropriate therapeutic strategies can be instituted where required, with specialist involvement if necessary. The lines of communication within a regional framework should be set out clearly, with the involvement of GPs intimately linked to the process of assessment. Clinical protocols should be clearly set out to minimise unnecessary repetition of investigations. Clinics should be structured so that patients are seen by the same clinician as far as possible and subspecialist input should be readily available if necessary. Information leaflets are a valuable adjunct to the smooth running of the clinic and suitably trained nursing staff are an integral part of the service. This allows treatment protocols to be planned on an individual basis and, linked to a sympathetic counselling service, serves the complex needs of an infertile population.

References

1. Royal College of Obstetricians and Gynaecologists. *The Initial Investigation and Management of the Infertile Couple.* Evidence-based Clinical Guidelines No. 2. London: RCOG Press; 1998.
2. Royal College of Obstetricians and Gynaecologists. The Management of Infertility in Secondary Care. Evidence-based Clinical Guidelines No. 3. London: RCOG Press; 1998.

3. National Collaborating Centre for Women's and Children's Health. *Fertility Assessment and Treatment for People with Fertility Problems*. London: RCOG Press; 2004.
4. Te Velde ER, Eijkemans R, Habbema HDF. Variation in couple fecundity and time to pregnancy, an essential concept in human reproduction. *Lancet* 2000; 355:1928–9.
5. Hamilton MPR. The initial assessment of the infertile couple. *Curr Obstet Gynaecol* 1992;2:2–7.
6. Oei SG, Helmerhorst FM, Keirse M. When is the postcoital test normal? A critical appraisal. *Hum Reprod* 1995;10:1711–14.

3 Male factor infertility

Introduction

A male factor problem is primarily responsible for up to 30% of cases of infertility and may be contributory in a further 20%. Assisted reproduction techniques, such as intracytoplasmic sperm injection (ICSI), have revolutionised its treatment and allowed men with severe oligozoospermia, and even some with azoospermia, to father their own children. Despite the success of such techniques, many of the underlying problems contributing to male infertility remain unexplored (see Chapter 8).

Aetiology

The diagnosis of male infertility is traditionally based on the identification of one or more abnormalities in semen parameters following laboratory analysis. Most men presenting with infertility cannot be given an explanation as to the cause of the problem, nor can an underlying pathology be identified. A study published by the World Health Organization (WHO) found no demonstrable cause in almost 50% of couples with male-factor infertility.[1] The distribution of diagnoses when male-factor subfertility was encountered in the WHO study are shown in Table 3.1.

Reports of falling sperm counts have yet to be linked with decreased fertility, although the effect of increased environmental estrogenic compounds is of concern due to the rising incidence of cryptorchidism and testicular cancer.

VARICOCOELE

A varicocoele is characterised by tortuous and engorged veins of the pampiniform plexus, which produce a swelling that feels like a 'bag of worms'. Its significance remains controversial, as it is relatively common, occurring in 5–20% of the general population and 10–40% of infertile men. Most varicocoeles are asymptomatic but some may cause dragging pain on the affected side. They are usually found coincidentally during

Table 3.1 Causes of male factor infertility (source: WHO survey, Rowe *et al.*[4])	
Cause	*Incidence (%)*
No demonstrable cause	48.8
Varicocoele	12.6
Idiopathic oligozoospermia	11.2
Accessory gland infection	6.9
Idiopathic teratozoospermia	5.9
Idiopathic asthenozoospermia	3.9
Isolated seminal plasma abnormalities	3.5
Suspected immunological subfertility	3.0
Congenital abnormalities	1.7
Systemic diseases	1.4
Sexual inadequacy	1.3
Obstructive azoospermia	0.9
Idiopathic necrozoospermia	0.8
Ejaculatory inadequacy	0.7
Hyperprolactinaemia	0.6
Iatrogenic causes	0.5
Karyotype abnormalities	0.1
Partial obstruction to ejaculatory duct	0.1
Retrograde ejaculation	0.1
Immotile cilia syndrome	< 1.0
Pituitary lesions	< 1.0
Gonadotrophin deficiency	< 1.0

investigation of a couple presenting with subfertility (Table 3.2) and are classified as primary (idiopathic) or secondary.

Primary or idiopathic varicocoeles are most common and thought to be due to:

- compression of the left renal vein between the aorta and the superior mesenteric artery (the nutcracker phenomenon)

Table 3.2	Clinical grade of varicocoele
Category	Description
Subclinical	No varicocoele at clinical examination but present on scrotal thermography or Doppler ultrasonography
Grade 1	No visible or palpable distension except on Valsalva manoeuvre
Grade 2	Intra-scrotal venous distension palpable, not visible
Grade 3	Distended venous plexus bulges through scrotal skin and easily palpable

- insufficiency of the valves in the left testicular vein, causing reflux of blood from the venocaval circulation down the left testicular vein to the pampiniform plexus of the testis and, through anastomosis, with the cremasteric plexus into the external iliac veins.

Secondary varicocoeles are rare and may occur due to obstruction of the left testicular vein by a growth like a hypernephroma along the renal veins. Characteristically, these varicocoeles do not decompress in the supine position.

Most varicocoeles are left-sided and associated with reduced testicular volume. The WHO suggests that there is an inverse relationship between semen quality and the presence and severity of varicocoeles, at least among the male partners of infertile couples and varicocoeles are associated with impaired testicular function and infertility. Surgical treatment of varicocoeles can involve ligation of the spermatic vein or embolisation. At the present time there is no evidence to suggest that surgical treatment of clinically detectable varicocoele in men with oligozoospermia will improve pregnancy rates.

HYPOGONADOTROPHIC HYPOGONADISM

This rare condition may be caused by hypothalamic or pituitary failure and can be congenital or acquired. Patients usually present with clinical evidence of androgen deficiency at around the time of puberty. However, adult onset (postpubertal) hypogonadotrophic hypogonadism may be recognised in males presenting with infertility due to trauma, tumour, chronic inflammatory lesions or iron overload.

In congenital hypogonadotrophic hypogonadism, a complete absence of gonadotrophin-releasing hormone (GnRH) results in the absence of secondary sexual development and total testicular failure, resulting in small, atrophic testes. However, males with a partial deficiency will have less profound manifestations of the disorder, with larger but yet underdeveloped testes. Most of these patients will have anosmia or hyposmia (Kallmann syndrome).

Low or undetectable levels of gonadotrophins (LH and FSH), which lead to lack of spermatogenesis and low testosterone levels, usually confirm the diagnosis.

COITAL DYSFUNCTION

Causes of coital dysfunction are shown in Table 3.3. Psychosexual dysfunction is an uncommon cause of male infertility, although it can accompany stress generated by prolonged investigations and treatment for infertility.

Table 3.3   Aetiology of coital dysfunction

Problem	Results from
Ejaculatory failure	Spinal cord injury
	Medical disorders:
	multiple sclerosis
	diabetes mellitus
	chronic renal failure
	Bladder-neck surgery
	Retroperitoneal lymph node dissection
Erectile or ejaculatory problems	Depression
	Alcohol abuse
	Medication:
	adrenergic blocking agents
	antihypertensive agents
	psychotrophic agents
	Psychosexual
Loss of libido and impotence	Hyperprolactinaemia due to:
	pituitary adenomas
	chronic renal failure
	idiopathic
	drug therapy
Retrograde ejaculation	Transurethral prostatectomy
	Retroperitoneal lymph-node dissection
	Diabetic neuropathy due to:
	injury to the lumbar sympathetic nerves
	damage to the neck of the bladder

The incidence of hyperprolactinaemia in impotent men ranges from 1–5%. Endocrine disorders such as androgen deficiency and hypothyroidism can also lead to coital dysfunction but usually present with the clinical manifestations of the specific disorder.

In patients with pituitary adenoma, symptoms such as impotence and loss of libido often precede other manifestations of the disorder. Imaging of the hypothalamo-pituitary axis is mandatory in all patients with sexual dysfunction and elevated prolactin levels.

Retrograde ejaculation is the propulsion of seminal fluid from the posterior urethra into the bladder. A diagnosis can be made by the absence of ejaculate (aspermia) and by the presence of a large number of spermatozoa in post-masturbatory urine.

IMMUNOLOGICAL CAUSES

Antisperm antibodies, which may be present in serum, seminal plasma or bound to spermatozoa have been associated with infertility, although their significance remains unclear. Antisperm antibodies are usually immunoglobulin G (IgG) or A (IgA) and can be bound to various sites on the spermatozoa (head, midpiece, tail or combinations thereof). Significant risk factors for the development of antisperm antibodies include vasectomy and infections such as epididymitis and orchitis.

Antisperm antibodies may have a detrimental affect on fertility by affecting sperm motility and causing:

- destruction of gametes
- acrosomal reaction abnormalities
- inhibition of zona pellucida binding
- prevention of embryo cleavage and early development of the embryo.

GENITAL TRACT INFECTION

Acute clinical infections of the genital tract (orchitis, epididymis, prostatovesiculitis or urethritis) may present with fever, pain and decreased sexual activity and may cause deterioration of semen quality or temporary obstruction of the genital tract. Gram-negative enterococci, chlamydia and gonococcus have all been associated with clinical infection. Transmission of acute infections to the female partner may lead to pelvic inflammatory disease and its sequelae, which includes tubal occlusion and infertility. Acute bacterial infections of the genital tract or sexually transmitted diseases can lead to infection of the accessory glands resulting in permanent structural damage and scarring, with obstruction to the outflow tract. Where such infection exists it should be treated with antibiotics. There is no evidence to suggest that antibiotic use will improve impaired male fertility. Symptomatic orchitis occurs in 27–30% of males over 11 years of age who are diagnosed with mumps. In 17% of cases it is bilateral. The prevalence of infertility after viral orchitis is unknown but impaired fertility occurs in bilateral orchitis due to seminiferous tubular atrophy and impairment of spermatogenesis.

GENITAL TRACT OBSTRUCTION

The most common cause of genital tract obstruction is iatrogenic following vasectomy. A post-infective cause should be suspected in men with azoospermia or oligozoospermia with normal-sized testes. The outcome following surgery depends on the skill of the surgeon and the site of obstruction. Epididymovasostomy is more successful when performed for a block in the caudal part of the epididymis than one in the capital part.

Ejaculatory duct obstruction is a rare cause of obstructive azoospermia and is commonly caused by congenital malformations, sometimes associated with abnormalities of the cystic fibrosis gene.

TESTICULAR MALDESCENT

Failure of the hypothalamic-pituitary-gonadal axis may be associated with failure of testicular descent, which occurs in 3–6% of males at birth.

As germ-cell degeneration and dysplasia resulting in irreversible testicular damage and infertility begins early in life, the abnormal position of the testis should be corrected by the end of the first year. There is also a five- to ten-fold increase in the risk of malignancy in the undescended testis. In addition to improving spermatogenesis, orchidopexy has beneficial psychological effects and prevents malignant change, trauma and torsion of the testes.

CHROMOSOMAL ABNORMALITIES

The most common chromosomal disorder affecting spermatogenesis is Klinefelter syndrome (47XXY). Fifteen percent of azoospermic men and 4% of oligozoospermic men have an abnormal chromosomal karyotype. An incidence of 2.2% of chromosomal abnormalities was detected in over 2000 men attending a male subfertility clinic over a 10-year period.

Other chromosomal abnormalities that may be found in the infertile male population include reciprocal X or Y autosomal translocations, as well as XYY and XX males. Males with azoospermia or severe oligo-zoospermia (less than 5 M/ml) should have a karyotype.

CHEMOTHERAPY, RADIOTHERAPY AND TOXINS

Treatment with certain drugs or exposure to radiation or chemicals can affect actively dividing germ cells causing defective spermatogenesis, which may be temporary or permanent.

Table 3.4 shows a list of drugs that interfere with spermatogenesis. Anabolic steroids used by some athletes can interfere with feedback to the pituitary, causing a reduction in gonadotrophin secretion. This results in testicular atrophy, which is reversible.

Cytotoxic drugs used for the treatment of testicular cancer, Hodgkin's disease, non-Hodgkin's lymphoma and leukaemia may have a deleterious affect on fertility. Cytotoxic treatment damages differentiating spermatogonia with most patients becoming azoospermic within eight weeks of commencing treatment. Alkylating agents may cause irreversible damage.

Exposure to radiation destroys germ cells with irreversible arrests of spermatogenesis, which invariably results in sterility.

Additionally, toxins in the workplace and environment may cause damage to the germ cells. A well-documented example is the chemical dibromochloropropane (DBCP), which caused azoospermia in 14 of 25 non-vasectomised men in a Californian pesticide factory.

Table 3.4 Therapeutic drugs interfering with male fertility (Rowe *et al.*[4])	
Drug	**Action**
Cancer chemotherapy	Alkylating agents cause irreversible damage.
Hormone treatment	High-dose corticosteroids, androgens, anti-androgens, estrogens and LH-releasing hormone agonist
Cimetidine	May competitively inhibit androgen effect on the receptor
Sulphasalazine	Can cause impairment of sperm quality by direct toxicity
Spironolactone	Antagonises the action of androgen in some tissue
Nitrofurantoin	May cause impairment of sperm quality by direct toxicity
Niradozole	May cause temporary depression of spermatogenesis in man
Colchicine	Causes depression of fertility by direct toxicity to spermatogenesis

IDIOPATHIC MALE INFERTILITY

Up to 50% of those with male factor subfertility have no demonstrable cause for their condition. A diagnosis of idiopathic infertility can only be made after all other causes of infertility have been excluded. Semen analysis may show varying degrees of abnormality and may be associated with elevated serum FSH, indicating failure of spermatogenesis.

KEY POINTS
- Varicocoeles are associated with impaired testicular function and infertility.
- Psychosexual dysfunction as a primary cause of male infertility is uncommon.
- Imaging of the hypothalamo-pituitary axis is mandatory in all patients with sexual dysfunction and elevated prolactin levels.
- About 70% of males have antisperm antibodies after vasectomy and this is of clinical importance if reversal is required.
- The most common cause of genital-tract obstruction is iatrogenic following vasectomy.
- Maldescended testis occurs in 3–6% of males at birth and should be corrected by the end of the first year.
- Males with azoospermia or severe oligozoospermia (less than 5 M/ml) should have a karyotype.
- Up to 50% of those with male factor subfertility have no demonstrable cause.

Clinical management

Both partners should be involved in the management. It is important to consider other factors, such as female age, duration of infertility and previous pregnancy when managing a couple with suboptimal semen parameters.

HISTORY AND EXAMINATION

A detailed history should be obtained from the male. It is important to enquire about previous infertility investigations undertaken in order to avoid repetition and save time and resources.

The male partner should be examined clinically, as described in Chapter 2.

Investigations

SEMEN ANALYSIS

Semen analysis should have been performed during initial investigations (see Chapter 2). This can be arranged in primary care. The RCOG evidence-based clinical guideline[2] on the initial investigation of the infertile couple recommends that: 'Laboratories that perform semen analysis should undertake this according to recognised WHO methodology. Laboratories should also perform internal quality control and belong to an external quality control scheme'. It is good practice to repeat the semen sample if the first specimen shows an abnormality.

If the semen analysis is abnormal or there is cause for concern in the history or clinical examination, further investigations of the male partner should be undertaken in a secondary or tertiary centre (see Chapter 2, Table 2.2 for normal values).

ENDOCRINE TESTS

Endocrine tests include:

- serum FSH
- serum testosterone
- prolactin.

Serum FSH

Serum FSH should be measured in the male partner with azoospermia or severe oligozoospermia (sperm density 5 M/ml or less). It has virtually replaced testicular biopsy in differentiating between an obstructive azoospermia (normal spermatogenesis) and non-obstructive or secretory azoospermia (failure of spermatogenesis).

In obstructive azoospermia, spermatogenesis is normal. In non-obstructive or secretory azoospermia there is failure of spermatogenesis.

FSH estimation may in addition give prognostic information in men prior to testicular biopsy if ICSI is being considered, although a high value does not totally exclude the possibility of sperm recovery.

Serum testosterone

Serum testosterone is only indicated if hypogonadism is suspected. Males with hypogonadism of hypothalamic or pituitary origin will have low FSH and low testosterone.

Prolactin

Virtually all men with hyperprolactinaemia have sexual dysfunction. It is mandatory to check for elevated prolactin levels in men complaining of loss of libido and impotence. Imaging of the hypothalamic–pituitary axis is indicated in males with high prolactin levels with no demonstrable cause to detect tumours such as prolactinoma, craniopharyngioma or tumours compressing the pituitary stalk.

It should be borne in mind that elevated prolactin levels might also occur in men on medication such as tranquillisers and sulpiride.

MICROBIOLOGICAL ASSESSMENT OF SEMEN

The biological significance of the presence of white blood cells in semen and asymptomatic subclinical infection is unclear. Many organisms are urethral contaminants of doubtful clinical significance. Semen culture should be performed in males with microscopic evidence of infections as well as those with symptoms of orchitis, epididymitis or prostatitis. Male partners of women with acute tubal disease should also be screened. Microbiological assessment may be indicated prior to intrauterine insemination although infective complications following intrauterine insemination are rare.

IMAGING OF THE GENITAL TRACT

Diagnostic tests of varicocoele

Varicocoele can be diagnosed by thermography, ultrasound with Doppler blood flow (higher false positive), radionuclide angiography (higher false negative) or retrograde venography. The last is the gold standard test, although it is invasive.

Scrotal ultrasound scan

Scrotal ultrasound is not performed routinely but should be undertaken if testicular tumours are suspected. In addition, an ultrasound may be helpful in detecting hydrocoeles and epididymal cysts and may be better than clinical examination.

Vasography

Vasography is performed in men with obstruction to the vas deferens and usually takes place in theatre prior to surgery, in order to detect the site of obstruction.

TESTICULAR BIOPSY

Testicular biopsy was initially used as a diagnostic tool to differentiate between obstructive and non-obstructive azoospermia and this has now been replaced by serum FSH measurements.

Testicular biopsy should be carried out only in tertiary centres, which have trained staff and facilities for sperm recovery and cryopreservation.[3] Sperm recovered during biopsy can be used for IVF, combined with ICSI, giving the opportunity for azoospermic men to father their own genetic offspring. Cryopreservation facilities should be available since sperm recovered may not be used for ICSI immediately.

Additionally, should sperm extraction not be carried out at the same time as the biopsy this may affect future attempts at sperm recovery due to the possibility of:

- reduction in testicular mass
- trauma causing devascularisation
- fibrosis
- an autoimmune response.

GENETIC STUDIES

Karyotyping/DNA analysis for Y chromosome microdeletions

Males with azoospermia or severe oligozoospermia should be karyotyped. Klinefelter syndrome is the most common chromosomal abnormality (46XXY) detected in this group.

Cystic fibrosis screen

The condition of congenital bilateral absence of the vas deferens (CBAVD) is, in the majority of patients, related to defects in the cystic fibrosis transmembrane conductance regulator (*CFTR*) gene. CBAVD is frequently associated with heterozygosity for the common cystic fibrosis gene (*DF 508*). A mutation analysis should be performed in males with CBAVD as well as the female partner, since the children have an increased risk of being born with cystic fibrosis and/or CBAVD.

Antisperm antibodies

Tests for antisperm antibodies are not routinely offered because there is no evidence of effective treatment to improve infertility.

Postcoital test

Current evidence suggests that the routine use of the postcoital test results in further investigations without significant improvement in terms of pregnancy rates. It is a poor predictor of fertility and it is difficult to justify this test as an essential procedure in standard infertility investigations.

- Female age, duration of infertility and history of previous pregnancy should be taken into account while interpreting the semen analysis for the individual couple.
- Clinical examination of the male is important and should be undertaken prior to any further investigations.
- Should semen analysis or clinical examination reveal abnormalities further investigations should be undertaken only in specialised centres.
- Serum FSH has virtually replaced testicular biopsy in differentiating between obstructive azoospermia and non-obstructive or secretory azoospermia.
- Antibiotic treatment is not currently recommended for asymptomatic genital tract infection.
- The postcoital test is a poor predictor of fertility and it is difficult to justify this test as an essential procedure in standard infertility investigations.

Treatment

GENERAL MANAGEMENT

The effect of age on male infertility is unclear. Alcohol consumption within the Department of Health's recommendations of three to four units a day is unlikely to affect fertility. However excessive alcohol intake is detrimental to semen quality. Men who smoke should be advised to stop smoking since there is an association between smoking and reduced semen quality (although the impact of this on male infertility is uncertain). A number of recreational and over the counter drugs (anabolic steroids and cocaine) interfere with male fertility.

Although there is an association between elevated scrotal temperature and reduced sperm quality it is uncertain whether wearing loose fitting underwear improves fertility.

MANAGEMENT OF VARICOCOELE

In the light of current evidence there is no justification for treating men with a clinically detectable varicocoele with normal sperm counts since this does not improve pregnancy rates. The evidence for treating oligozoospermic men is uncertain and benefit is far from clear.

The surgical procedure that is usually undertaken is ligation of the spermatic vein above the inguinal ligament at the internal inguinal ring. Only occasionally is a local excision indicated in cases where ligation leaves a group of tortuous varicosities. Alternatively, testicular vein embolisation can be undertaken under radiological guidance (Figure 3.1).

MANAGEMENT OF GONADOTROPHIN DEFICIENCY

Hypogonadotrophic hypogonadism is one of the few conditions in men that can be treated successfully with complete restoration of steroidogenesis and spermatogenesis (Table 3.5).

Treatment with exogenous gonadotrophins or GnRH therapy can result in effective spermatogenesis in 70–90% of men, who become fertile even with sperm counts well below normal limits. Once fertility has been achieved, treatment can be substituted with testosterone in the form of oral, injectable or implant.

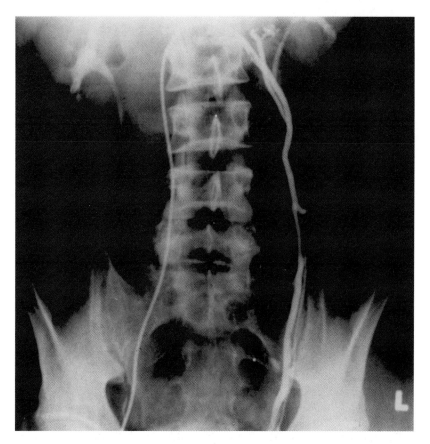

Figure 3.1   X-ray of embolism of left-sided varicocoele

Table 3.5 Summary of management of gonadotrophic deficiency

Treatment	Deficiency	Action	Administration
hCG (source of LH activity)	Acquired HH	Stimulates Leydig cells to produce testosterone	Intramuscular injection
hCG + hMG (source of FSH)	Acquired/prepubertal HH	As above and causes maturation and proliferation of the germinal cells; stimulates spermatogenesis	Intramuscular injection
hCG +FSH-HP (better tolerated)	Acquired/prepubertal HH	Effective in stimulating spermatogenesis and steroidogenesis	Self-administered subcutaneously over months/years to achieve maximum testicular size and spermatogenesis
Pulsatile GnRH therapy	HH of hypothalamic origin	Stimulation of the pituitary and testis; stimulates spermatogenesis	Battery-driven portable infusion pump; administers set dose subcutaneously (worn continuously approx. l year)
Dopamine agonists (bromocriptine)	HH due to prolactinoma (causing hyperprolactinaemia)	Normalises serum prolactin levels, LH secretion begins, testosterone levels normalise, restoration of potency and fertility	5–10 mg/day in divided doses

HH = hypogonadotrophic hypogonadism

MANAGEMENT OF EJACULATORY PROBLEMS

Counselling forms an important part in the management of couples with psychosexual dysfunction. Various methods of semen procurement such as external vibratory massage, intrathecal injection of neostigmine, direct aspiration of sperm from the vas and electroejaculation have been tried in men with erectile and ejaculatory dysfunction. Rectal probe electroejaculation has become an accepted method to procure sperm with successful sperm recovery in over 80% of cases. Sperm procured from electroejaculation can be used for intrauterine insemination (IUI) or IVF.

The sperm quality following electroejaculation is usually poor, with a high sperm count and usually normal morphology but low motility. The possible aetiologies for low sperm motility include:

- stasis of seminal fluid
- testicular hyperthermia
- recurrent urinary tract infections
- antisperm antibodies
- urinary contamination due to retrograde ejaculation
- (possibly) effects of heat and electric current generated by electroejaculation.

This can probably be overcome with IVF and IVF/ICSI. At present it is not possible to estimate pregnancy rates with a combination of electroejaculation and assisted reproductive technology in view of the small numbers of patients.

The efficacy of medical treatment of retrograde ejaculation is disputable since no randomised controlled trials have been conducted to determine efficacy. Medical treatment for reversal of retrograde ejaculation facilitates antegrade ejaculation by stimulating peristalsis in the vas deferens and closing the bladder neck. This may be achieved by either increasing sympathetic tone at the bladder neck or by decreasing parasympathetic activity. Drugs used are shown in Table 3.6.

Table 3.6 Drugs included in treatment of retrograde ejaculation	
Type of drug	**Preparation**
Alpha-adrenergic agonists	Phenylpropanolamine hydrochloride 25 mg orally twice daily
	Oxedrine 15–60 mg in a single intravenous dose
Anticholinergics	Brompheniramine maleate 8 mg twice daily
	Imipramine in a daily dose of 25–50 mg

Selective phosphodiesterase type 5 inhibitors such as sildenafil (Viagra®, Pfizer) and vardenafil (Levitra®, Bayer) are effective treatments for erectile dysfunction. Other available therapy includes:

- implants
- intracavernosal injection
- intraurethral pellets
- vacuum devices
- sex therapy.

The pathway for sexual arousal and stimulation leading to erection is the production of cyclic guanosine monophosphate (cGMP) in the corpus cavernosum, which relaxes the smooth muscle and causes blood to fill the corpora. Sildenafil specifically inhibits the isoenzyme cGMP specific phosphodiesterase type five, which is responsible for the breakdown of cGMP in the corpus cavernosum. Hence, it produces sexual arousal or stimulation similar to a 'natural' erectile response. Although orgasmic function, satisfaction with intercourse and overall sexual function is improved, it has no effect on sexual drive.

Sildenafil is administered in a dose of 30–60 mg. Common adverse effects include headache, flushing, dyspepsia, nasal congestion and transient disturbance of colour discrimination. It can cause priapism and can potentiate the hypotensive effect of nitrates.

IMMUNOLOGICAL INFERTILITY MANAGEMENT

Immunological male factor infertility refers to the presence of anti-sperm antibodies in the seminal fluid or bound to spermatozoa. It accounts for about 3% of male factor infertility. The majority of trials evaluating the role of steroids in the treatment of antisperm antibodies are uncontrolled or methodologically flawed in other ways. Adverse effects of steroids include dyspepsia, facial flushing, bloating, irritability, skin rashes and Cushingoid appearance with rare serious complications such as bilateral aseptic necrosis of the hip and the risk of severe chickenpox in an unexposed individual. Owing to the potentially serious adverse effects of steroids and conflicting evidence of benefit, their use can only be recommended in the context of further research. Patients with high levels of IgA or IgG antibodies should be directly referred for ICSI.

MANAGEMENT OF GENITAL TRACT OBSTRUCTION

Reported success rates for vasectomy reversal vary from 17–82%. Factors influencing success rates include:

- type of vasectomy performed
- type of reversal
- surgical technique (macro- or microsurgery)
- presence of other pathology such as varicocoeles or antisperm antibodies
- the experience and skill of the surgeon
- time since vasectomy.

The last two factors are the most important, surgical skill being important for microsurgical techniques.

The longer the time interval from vasectomy to reversal, the lower the chance of a successful pregnancy, because of the risk of secondary epididymal obstruction.

The most cost-effective approach to the treatment of post-vasectomy infertility is microsurgical reversal. This treatment also has the highest chance of resulting in delivery of a child for a single intervention with a delivery rate of 47%, whereas after one cycle of sperm retrieval and ICSI the delivery rate is around 30%. Vasectomy reversal has, in addition, added advantages over ICSI, including the possibility of further pregnancies without further intervention, conception following normal intercourse and avoidance of ovarian hyperstimulation and multiple pregnancy.

Reversal of vasectomy should be the first line of treatment in men wishing fertility after vasectomy and at present microsurgical epididymal sperm aspiration and ICSI should be reserved for failed surgery or in men where surgical reconstruction is not feasible.

Obstructive lesions of the genital tract are not a common cause of infertility and reconstructive surgical treatment should only be undertaken by trained surgeons with microsurgical skills in specialist centres with facilities for microsurgery, sperm retrieval and cryostorage.

EMPIRICAL TREATMENT, INCLUDING TREATMENT NOT YET SHOWN TO BE EFFECTIVE

Gonadotrophins

Gonadotrophins, human chorionic gonadotrophin (hCG) and human menopausal gonadotrophin (hMG) have been used successfully in males with hypogonadotrophic hypogonadism and this has led to its use in idiopathic male infertility. However, there is no evidence to recommend gonadotrophin treatment for idiopathic male infertility.

Gonadotrophin-releasing hormone

GnRH has been used in males with subnormal semen parameters but did not improve semen parameters in idiopathic male infertility.

Androgens

Testosterone is required for normal spermatogenesis. This led to the use of androgens (e.g. mesterolone) in idiopathic male infertility but there is no evidence to support the effectiveness of this treatment. Testosterone exerts a negative feedback effect on the pituitary–gonadal axis, suppressing FSH and LH secretion and thereby adversely affecting spermatogenesis. Oral doses of testosterone required to achieve serum levels equivalent to intra-testicular levels can cause hepatotoxicity.

Bromocriptine

Bromocriptine has been shown to be beneficial in men with hyperprolactinaemia, with or without hypogonadotrophic hypogonadism. In normo-gonadotrophic males, it does not reduce prolactin levels and does not improve semen parameters or fertility.

Anti-estrogens

Clomifene or tamoxifen have been used commonly for idiopathic male infertility. Many observational studies have shown apparent improvements in sperm concentration and/or motility as well as pregnancy rates. However, a review of randomised studies provides no proof of effectiveness of anti-estrogens.

Kallikrein

Kallikrein is a glycoprotein that causes release of kinins from kininogens. Although the mechanism of action of kallikrein is unclear, it has been suggested that a local increase in kinins at the testicular level influences spermatogenesis. In vitro studies have shown that kallikrein assists sperm motility and improves cervical mucus penetration. Following these observations kallikrein was used in the treatment of idiopathic male infertility. However, recent randomised controlled studies have not shown any demonstrable benefits and the drug should not be used.

Antioxidants

Antioxidants such as glutathione, vitamin E and vitamin C may improve semen parameters. However, at this stage no recommendations can be given for the use of antioxidants for the treatment of male infertility and this mode of treatment requires further evaluation.

Mast-cell blockers

Initial results for the use of a mast-cell blocker (tranilast) in the treatment of severe oligozoospermia have been promising. This treatment requires further evaluation.

Alpha blockers

Bunazosin has also been shown to improve sperm concentration and motility although there was no difference in pregnancy rates. Again, further studies are needed to evaluate the effectiveness of this treatment.

Assisted reproduction

SUPEROVULATION AND IUI

IUI, with or without ovarian stimulation, improves the relative odds of pregnancy in the presence of abnormalities of semen parameters. The actual pregnancy rates remain low (4–6%). Thus, while the use of insemination may be justified the results cannot be compared with those following ICSI.

ICSI

Men with severe sperm abnormalities or non-obstructive azoospermia now have the possibility of fathering their own children by means of ICSI or microsurgical sperm retrieval followed by ICSI (Chapter 8).

DONOR INSEMINATION

The use of unstimulated cycles should be considered the first line of treatment to avoid multiple pregnancy. While the use of gonadotrophin stimulation will increase pregnancy rates, multiple pregnancy rates are likely to be much higher. An overall pregnancy rate of 10% per cycle for unstimulated donor insemination cycles should be anticipated.

KEY POINTS
- The significance of a varicocoele in male infertility is controversial, but treatment is unlikely to be helpful.
- Gonadotrophins for hypogonadotrophic hypogonadism and bromocriptine for hyperprolactinaemia are effective treatments.
- The efficacy of medical treatment of retrograde ejaculation is disputable.
- Systemic steroids cannot be currently recommended for immunological infertility.
- Vasectomy reversal should be considered the first line of treatment in men requesting reversal of sterilisation.
- ICSI is an effective treatment but exposes the female to the hazards of assisted reproduction and does not cure the underlying male anomaly.

Table 3.7   Prevention of infertility

- Surgical treatment (orchidopexy) is indicated by the end of the first year in males with testicular maldescent should endocrine therapy fail, to prevent irreversible damage.

- Infections, particularly chlamydia, should be screened for and treated appropriately to prevent upper tract infection, which may lead to pelvic inflammatory disease and its sequelae.

- Health advice regarding smoking and alcohol consumption should be given.

- Patients should avoid using drugs that cause deterioration of semen parameters and use alternative drugs when available.

- Elective cryopreservation of sperm prior to radiotherapy or chemotherapy should be offered.

Prevention

Methods of preventing male infertility are shown in Table 3.7.

References

1. World Health Organization. The influence of varicocoele on parameters of fertility in a large group of men presenting to infertility clinics. *Fertil Steril* 1992;57:1289–93.
2. Royal College of Obstetricians and Gynaecologists. *The Initial Investigation and Management of the Infertile Couple*. Evidence-based Clinical Guideline No. 2. London: RCOG Press; 1998.
3. Royal College of Obstetricians and Gynaecologists. *The Management of Infertility in Secondary Care*. Evidence-based Clinical Guideline No. 3. London: RCOG Press; 1998.
4. Rowe PJ, Comhaire FH, Hargreave TB, Mellows HJ. *WHO Manual for the Standardised Investigation and Diagnosis of the Infertile Couple*. Cambridge: Cambridge University Press; 1993.

Further reading

National Collaborating Centre for Women's and Children's Health. *Fertility: Assessment and Treatment for People with Fertility Problems*. London: RCOG Press; 2004.

4 Disorders of ovulation

Introduction

Ovulatory dysfunction is the principal cause in about one-fifth of all infertile couples, with quoted incidences varying from 10% to 50%. Despite advances in the management of anovulation, there continues to be a disparity between rates of successful ovulation induction and pregnancy. This may be explained by inadequate investigation of other factors contributing to infertility (Chapter 3). There are also iatrogenic problems associated with ovulation induction, particularly ovarian hyperstimulation syndrome (OHSS), multiple gestation and a putative risk of ovarian malignancy with repeated ovarian stimulation. The aim of current treatment regimens is not only to achieve higher pregnancy rates, but also to minimise treatment related complications.

Classification of ovulation disorders

Ovulation disorders can be classified on the basis of their anatomical site in the hypothalamic–pituitary–ovarian axis.

OVARY

Causes of intrinsic ovarian failure include:

- genetic
- Turner syndrome (46XO)
- Turner mosaic (XO,XX)
- XX gonadal agenesis
- autoimmune ovarian failure
- pelvic radiotherapy
- chemotherapy
- premature menopause.

HYPOTHALAMUS

GnRH regulates gonadotrophin secretion from the pituitary. The ovary may be affected by abnormalities of GnRH secretion from the hypothalamus. This happens in cases of hyperprolactinaemia and Kallmann syndrome, the latter characterised by a lack of GnRH, anosmia and other congenital abnormalities. Weight loss, excessive exercise and stress may also result in altered GnRH secretion.

PITUITARY

Disorders of the pituitary itself can result in gonadotrophin deficiency. These include tumour necrosis and thrombosis of the pituitary. Sheehan syndrome is the result of postpartum pituitary necrosis secondary to hypovolaemia associated with severe postpartum haemorrhage.

HYPOTHALAMIC–PITUITARY DYSFUNCTION

Hypothalamic–pituitary dysfunction can result in oligo-/anovulation, as in polycystic ovary syndrome (PCOS), which is associated with hyperinsulinaemia and hyperandrogenaemia.

The WHO classification of ovulatory disorders is shown in Table 4.1.

Diagnosis

Treatment of anovulation depends upon correct identification of the underlying problem. Regular menstruation (26–36 day cycles) is strongly suggestive of ovulation but not conclusive. A midluteal serum progesterone level (day 21 in a 28-day cycle) of 30 nmol/l or above is accepted as confirmatory (see Chapter 2). With irregular cycles, serial progesterone tracking (weekly) until the next menstrual cycle may be necessary. In women with very irregular or infrequent periods, treatment may be indicated irrespective of proven ovulation.

In women with primary amenorrhoea and absent sexual development, investigations should include serum FSH and LH. Low levels (less than 5 iu/l) could indicate a hypogonadotrophic hypogonadism or an intracranial lesion. Levels over 30 iu/l would provoke the necessity for karyotyping to look for Turner syndrome or its variants, XX gonadal agenesis, 46XY gonadal agenesis or testicular enzymatic failure. Patients in whom a Y chromosome is detected should be advised that they have a 30% risk of malignancy and gonadectomy should be discussed. Women with primary amenorrhoea and normal sexual characteristics need a detailed clinical examination and investigations to rule out outflow tract obstruction. The absence of a uterus and/or vagina in these

Table 4.1   WHO classification of ovulatory deficiencies

Group	Type of deficiency	Ovulatory dysfunction (%)	Characteristics
I	Hypothalamic pituitary failure (hypothalamic amenorrhoea or hypogonadotrophic hypogonadism)	10	Low-basal gonadotrophins, normal prolactin and estrogen deficiency with a failure to bleed after a progestational challenge. Includes amenorrhoea related to stress and weight loss, Kallmann syndrome, isolated gonadotrophin deficiency and idiopathic hypogonadotrophic hypogonadism.
II	Hypothalamic pituitary dysfunction	85	Normal gonadotrophins and estrogen levels with anovulatory oligo-/amenorrhoea. PCOS is the predominant example here, being present in 80–90% of women with oligomenorrhoea and in 30% with amenorrhoea.
III	Ovarian failure	4–5	High levels of gonadotrophins with hypogonadism and low estrogen levels. Includes premature ovarian failure, ovarian failure due to genetic, autoimmune, cytotoxic radiotherapy/chemotherapy, etc.

women would call for karyotyping to detect androgen insensitivity (testicular feminisation syndrome). Rarely, primary amenorrhoea is due to PCOS, a resistant ovary or hyperprolactinaemia.

Serum prolactin estimation is indicated in women with symptoms of oligomenorrhoea or amenorrhoea (primary or secondary), galactorrhoea or a pituitary tumour. Although women with subfertility are no more likely than the general population to have subclinical thyroid disease,[1] there is a view (PCOS Consensus Workshop Group) that performing thyroid function tests in the hyperandrogenic, oligo-/anovulatory woman need not be discouraged.

Oligo-/amenorrhoea, especially when associated with weight gain, acne or hirsutism, would call for investigations to confirm PCOS (discussed further below).

In women with a history of amenorrhoea and weight loss or stress, a low FSH and LH level (less than 5 iu/l) will confirm hypogonadotrophic hypogonadism. High FSH and low oestradiol levels in the presence of amenorrhoea is confirmatory of ovarian failure. Other investigations to detect autoimmune problems include a full blood count, tests for rheumatoid factor, antinuclear antibodies, a thyroid screen with auto-antibody testing and tests for adrenal function.

POLYCYSTIC OVARY SYNDROME

PCOS is characterised by ovulatory dysfunction and hyperandroge-naemia. While the pathogenesis is poorly understood, the primary defect is thought to be insulin resistance. Chronic hyperinsulinaemia leads to overproduction of ovarian androgens and decrease in serum sex hormone-binding globulin levels, leading to increased bioavailability of free testosterone. The high androgen levels lead to anovulation/ oligo-ovulation, menstrual disturbances and hirsutism.

The revised diagnostic criteria[1] of PCOS include the presence of two of: oligo- and/or anovulation; clinical and/or biochemical signs of hyperan-drogenism; polycystic ovaries; in the absence of the following: congeni-tal adrenal hyperplasia, androgen secreting tumours, Cushing syndrome, hyperprolactinaemia, thyroid dysfunction.

The primary clinical marker of hyperandrogenism is hirsutism, bearing in mind that the assessment of hirsutism can be subjective, and it may be less prevalent in adolescents and hyperandrogenic women of East Asian origin. Other clinical features are acne and androgenic alopecia. High free testosterone and/or free testosterone (free androgen) index (FAI) are the biochemical indicators of PCOS. Some women with PCOS may have iso-lated elevations in dehydroepiandrosterone sulphate (DHEA-S). There is paucity of data on the role of androstenedione measurements in PCOS and currently its routine assessment is not recommended.

The definition of polycystic-appearing ovaries on scan includes the presence of 12 or more peripheral follicles in each ovary, measuring 2–9 mm in diameter, and/or increased ovarian volume (greater than 10 ml). Ovarian volume is calculated using the formula for a prolate ellipsoid (0.5 × length × width × thickness) and is a good surrogate for the quantification of stromal volume, which is increased and also appears more echogenic in PCOS. The distribution of follicles is not included in the definition and only one ovary fitting the description is sufficient for the diagnosis (Figure 4.1).

Ultrasound scans (preferably vaginal, especially in women who are obese) should be performed in oligo-/anovulatory women either at random or between days 3 and 5 after a progestogen-induced bleed. In

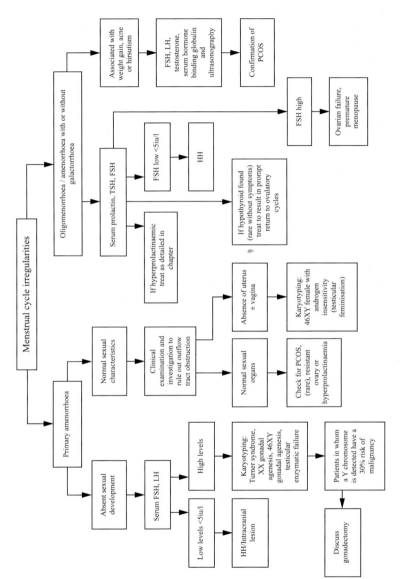

Figure 4.1 Investigations used in the diagnosis of ovulatory disorders

regularly menstruating women, it should be performed in the early follicular phase (days 3–5). If there is a follicle greater than 10 mm or a
corpus luteal cyst, the scan should be repeated at a time of ovarian qui-
escence, in order to calculate ovarian volume and to assess for the presence of cysts that might need further investigation.

Insulin resistance is a common feature of PCOS, seen in 50–80% of
women with PCOS who are obese and those who are not. However, currently there is no clinical test that has been validated for detecting
insulin resistance in these women. Criteria for defining a metabolic syndrome are centripetal obesity (waist circumference greater than 88 cm),
hypertension ($\geq$ 130/$\geq$ 85), fasting hyperglycaemia (6–7 mmol/l) and/
or an increase in 2-hour glucose levels after a 75-g glucose load
(7.7–11 mmol/l), an increase in triglycerides ($\geq$ 1.7 mmol/l) and a
decrease in high-density lipoproteins ($\leq$ 1.3 mmol/l).

Elevated LH levels are seen in about 60% and altered LH/FSH ratios in
up to 95% of women with PCOS (after exclusion of ovulation). The role
of elevated LH levels on oocyte maturation and fertilisation, and on
pregnancy and miscarriage rates, is controversial and contradictory.
Serum LH and FSH levels, although useful as secondary parameters
(especially in the lean woman with oligo-/anovulation) are not considered necessary for the clinical diagnosis of PCOS.

Women with PCOS are at three to seven times the risk of developing
type 2 diabetes, especially if they are obese, anovulatory or have a family
history of type 2 diabetes. There are some epidemiological data to
suggest that these women might be at increased risk of cardiovascular
disease (due to dyslipidaemia) and endometrial cancer (due to unop-
posed estrogen exposure of the endometrium). It is thus good clinical
practice to recommend treatment with progestogens to induce a withdrawal bleed at least every 3–4 months. It may also be useful to screen
pregnant women with PCOS for gestational diabetes.

Treatment options: considerations

Before embarking on treatment for ovulation induction, the following
should be considered:

- relevant investigations to make an accurate diagnosis
- selection of the most appropriate treatment
- counselling of the patient regarding potential risks of:
  - OHSS
  - multiple pregnancy
  - possibility of fetal reduction
  - putative risk of ovarian cancer

- ovulation induction; should be undertaken only in the presence of adequate monitoring facilities, including free availability of ultrasonography and endocrinology
- protocols for cancelling cycles to prevent multiple gestations and OHSS
- exclusion of coexistent male factor problems (i.e. semen analysis: motile sperm count of at least 5 million/ejaculate)
- tubal patency, using hysterosalpingography in women at low risk of tubal disease; a laparoscopy and dye transit test is useful if more detailed pelvic examination is desired or where endometriosis or pelvic adhesions are suspected.
- Formal tubal evaluation may be deferred in women at low risk of tubal disease until six treatment cycles with clomifene have been completed.
- General preconception advice includes folate supplements, smoking, rubella status and weight loss or gain, especially with a BMI over 25 or less than 20 kg/m^2.

Treatment options in WHO group II ovulatory dysfunction (mainly PCOS) include:

- weight loss
- insulin sensitising drugs, such as metformin:
  - used alone
  - used in combination with clomifene, gonadotrophins
- anti-estrogens (clomifene citrate, tamoxifen):
  - used alone
  - used in combination with dexamethasone, hMG or hCG
- gonadotrophins (hMG, purified FSH and recombinant FSH):
  - used alone
  - used in combination with GnRH agonists and antagonists
- low-dose gonadotrophin therapy
- aromatase inhibitors (letrozole)
- laparoscopic ovarian drilling.

Weight loss and lifestyle modification

Central obesity and increased BMI are major determinants of insulin resistance and hyperandrogenaemia in PCOS. Successful treatment of obesity has been shown to reverse endocrine abnormalities associated with PCOS and to encourage spontaneous cyclic ovarian activity and response to ovulation induction agents. Apart from general improvement of health, this approach leads to lower ovarian hyperstimulation and miscarriage rates and higher pregnancy rates. A reduction in 5–10% in body weight has been shown to restore reproductive function in 55–100% women within 6 months of weight reduction. While lifestyle changes are difficult to maintain, women seeking pregnancy are highly motivated, making this a reasonable first-line intervention in women with subfertility who are obese.

Insulin-sensitising agents

Because of the role of hyperinsulinaemia in PCOS, insulin-sensitising agents have been used to reverse the endocrinological and clinical features of PCOS. The most widely used agent in PCOS is metformin, an orally administered biguanide used in type 2 diabetes mellitus. It enhances insulin sensitivity in the liver, where it inhibits hepatic glucose production, and in the peripheral tissues, where it increases the uptake and utilisation of glucose in muscle. It does not provoke hyperinsulinaemia and therefore carries no risk of hypoglycaemia. Newer insulin-sensitising agents include the thiazolidinedione group of drugs, which include troglitazone (now withdrawn because of hepatotoxicity) and rosiglitazone and pioglitazone.

A systematic review suggests that there is little evidence that metformin causes weight loss, but it does reverse some of the metabolic features in PCOS (reducing fasting insulin and low-density lipoprotein concentrations).[2] Used as a sole agent in PCOS, it resulted in ovulation in 46% of women on metformin, as compared with 24% receiving placebo. When used in combination with clomifene, ovulation was noted in 76%, as compared with 42% receiving clomifene alone. Therefore metformin appears to be successful as pre-treatment and co-treatment with clomifene, perhaps by sensitising follicles to FSH.

Adverse effects of metformin include nausea, vomiting and gastrointestinal disturbance. It is contraindicated in the presence of renal impairment because of the danger of lactic acidosis. While it is not known to be teratogenic, the current practice is to stop its use when pregnancy is confirmed, as sufficient data for its safety in pregnancy are lacking. There are also limited data on the safety of its long-term use in young women. It is associated with decreased absorption of vitamin B12.

While, thus far, metformin has been mainly used in women with PCOS who have not responded to clomifene, there is a growing trend towards its use as a first-line drug treatment where diet and lifestyle modifications have not been effective.[2] Metformin also carries fewer risks of multiple pregnancy and OHSS as compared with other ovulation induction agents. The recommended starting dose is 500 mg twice a day with meals, increasing to 500 mg three times daily. The dose can be increased to 1 g twice daily, if tolerated. In the absence of a pregnancy within 6–12 months of metformin use alone, clomifene could be added. Renal and hepatic function should be checked annually in women on long-term metformin.

While there is some evidence that outcomes may be improved when metformin pre-treatment is used with gonadotrophin ovulation induction and IVF, there is not enough evidence for this at present and this is not currently recommended as routine practice.

Anti-estrogens

CLOMIFENE CITRATE

Clomifene citrate has been in use since the 1960s and remains the most commonly prescribed drug for induction of ovulation. It accounts for two-thirds of all the fertility drugs used currently. It is similar in structure to the synthetic estrogen, diethylstilbestrol.

MECHANISM OF ACTION

Clomifene binds to estrogen receptors in the hypothalamus exerting a weak biological estrogen-like effect. The hypothalamic–pituitary axis is blinded to endogenous estrogen levels, which are falsely perceived to be low. This reduces the negative feedback caused by estrogen, resulting in an increase in GnRH secretion from the hypothalamus. This in turn leads to a rise in FSH production, which stimulates follicular recruitment and growth.

An intact hypothalamo–pituitary axis is essential for the effects of clomifene. It is most useful in normogonadotrophic oligo-/amenorrhoeic women (mainly PCOS, WHO Group II). Women with hypogonadotrophic hypogonadism (WHO Group I) and those with ovarian tissue not capable of responding to gonadotrophins (WHO Group III) are not suitable for clomifene.

TREATMENT REGIMENS

Treatment regimens should be started with the lowest dose that could achieve ovulation. This is generally assumed to be 50 mg taken orally every day for 5 days from day 2 to day 6 of the menstrual cycle. Occasionally, in women exceptionally sensitive to clomifene, a 25-mg dose may be adequate. In amenorrhoeic women, once a pregnancy is ruled out and E_2 and progesterone levels are basal, treatment may be started with or without a progesterone-induced withdrawal bleed.

The patient is assessed for adverse effects and ovulation checked with a luteal phase progesterone estimation. Because of the risk of multiple pregnancy and the variable response of women to different doses of clomifene, it is necessary to monitor at least the first clomifene cycle with ultrasonography. If there is no response to 50 mg, the dose is increased to 100 mg daily and then to 150 mg. The couple is advised to have intercourse every other day at least, from day 9 or 10 of the cycle for at least a week.

ADVERSE DRUG REACTIONS

Adverse effects of clomifene are not dose related and can occur even with the lowest doses used. The usual problems are hot flushes (in about 10%), with a small minority (2%) of women complaining of abdominal distension, pain, nausea, vomiting, breast tenderness, headache and reversible hair loss. Clomifene also has a mydriatic action and about 1.5% of women have blurred vision and scotomas. These symptoms disappear once the drug is stopped. Significant ovarian enlargement can occur in about 5% of patients, but full-blown OHSS is rare. The incidence of multiple pregnancy is about 7–10% and mainly involves twins. Higher order pregnancies have also been reported. This highlights the necessity for ultrasound monitoring with clomifene.

EFFECTIVENESS

In properly selected women, clomifene seems highly effective in achieving ovulation in 70–80% of normogonadotrophic women. A pregnancy rate per ovulatory cycle of 20–25% has been described and could be due to coexisting tubal disease, endometriosis and male factors. Doses over 100 mg may lower pregnancy rates due to anti-estrogenic effects on cervical mucus and endometrium. The cumulative pregnancy rate over 6 months of clomifene use approaches 60–70%. The incidence of congenital anomalies is not increased, although the miscarriage rate is 20–25%.

There is evidence to suggest that cumulative pregnancy rates in women who ovulate with clomifene and have no other infertility problems continue to rise after six cycles but begin to plateau by about ten treatment cycles. Therefore, treatment up to 12 cycles is recommended.

The need for monitoring with ultrasonography during clomifene treatment may mean that clomifene should be prescribed by a specialist clinic.

TAMOXIFEN

Tamoxifen is a drug that is similar to clomifene, with similar actions. It appears to be as effective in inducing ovulation as clomifene but data from randomised trials are limited.

COMBINATION OF CLOMIFENE AND DEXAMETHASONE

In women with high circulating levels of androgens who are resistant to clomifene, dexamethasone 0.5 mg at night throughout the cycle has been found to decrease the adrenal contribution to the circulating androgens. This may result in better responsiveness to clomifene. However, weight gain due to medium- to long-term glucocorticoid steroid therapy in women with PCOS has to be balanced against any potential advantages.

COMBINATION OF CLOMIFENE WITH HCG

Human chorionic gonadotrophin in doses of 5000–10 000 iu has been used to induce ovulation in clomifene treatment cycles where ovulation cannot be confirmed by serum progesterone levels despite visualisation of a dominant follicle. Ultrasound monitoring is needed to ensure that hCG is administered when the leading follicle is of preovulatory size (greater than 17 mm).

Gonadatrophins

The main indication for treatment with gonadotrophins (hMG, purified FSH, recombinant FSH) in WHO group II patients is failure to conceive with clomifene with or without metformin.

Human menopausal gonadotrophin is prepared from extracts of urine from postmenopausal women. The ratio of FSH to LH is one to one and the commercial preparation contains 75 iu each of FSH and LH (e.g. Pergonal®, Humegon®). It is administered by deep intramuscular injection. Purified FSH (e.g. Metrodin®) is predominantly FSH with an FSH to LH ratio of approximately 75 to 1. It may be administered intramuscularly or subcutaneously. Recombinant FSH (e.g. Puregon®, Gonal F®) produced through genetic engineering has a high purity and lacks LH. These preparations are free of the contamination by proteins that is seen in preparations from urinary extracts. They are administered subcutaneously.

There is, at present, little evidence to suggest that purified or recombinant FSH is more effective than hMG. However, recombinant FSH is associated with a reduction in the total dosage of FSH and a shorter duration of treatment.

TREATMENT REGIMEN

Follicular stimulation is achieved by daily hMG/FSH injections. The number and size of developing follicles is monitored using transvaginal ultrasonography of the ovaries and circulating estradiol levels. The dose of hMG/FSH may need to be modified depending on estradiol (E_2) levels and the ovarian follicular response. When the dominant follicle is at least 17 mm, 5000–10 000 iu of hCG is administered subcutaneously. The woman is advised to have intercourse the day of the hCG injection and, if possible, for the next 2 days.

The aim of ovulation induction is to induce unifollicular ovulation with minimal occurrence of OHSS and multiple pregnancies. When E_2 levels are over 5500 pmol/l and/or more than three follicles over 17 mm are seen, hCG should be withheld and the cycle cancelled to minimise the above mentioned risks.

EFFECTIVENESS

Cumulative success rates of approximately 40–50% in WHO group II patients have been reported.

ADVERSE EFFECTS

Miscarriage rates associated with gonadotrophin ovulation induction are between 25% and 30%. There is no increase in congenital malformations. The risk of ectopic gestations is higher and this may be due to the multiple oocytes and the high hCG levels. The rate of serious OHSS is about 1–2%. The major concern is the high multiple pregnancy rate which is about 15–20%.

LOW-DOSE GONADOTROPHIN REGIMENS

Women with polycystic ovaries are at a higher risk of developing OHSS (5%) and multiple pregnancies (34%) with gonadotrophin therapy.[3] The use of a low-dose step-up gonadotrophin regimen may reduce this risk; hMG/FSH is started at a dose of 75 iu daily for up to 14 days, then increased to 112.5 iu for another 7 days if there is no ovarian response, then to 150 iu and so on, until the maximum dose of 225 iu daily is reached. Once ovarian activity is seen, the same dose is continued until follicular maturation is seen on scan and then the ovulatory trigger of hCG given. In 100 women treated with this protocol, there was a cumulative pregnancy rate of 55% after six treatment cycles with no case of severe OHSS; 73% of all cycles were uniovular, with only two multiple pregnancies. Low-dose regimens reduce the serious risks of OHSS and multiple pregnancy.

AROMATASE INHIBITORS

These are drugs that suppress the negative feedback effect of estrogen on the hypothalamic–pituitary system by reducing its secretion by the ovaries. This causes a rise in FSH levels leading to follicular development. Letrozole, a third-generation aromatase inhibitor, has been used in anovulatory women with PCOS who are resistant to clomifene with some success. Initial studies on a small sample of women suggest that a dose of 2.5 mg on days 3–7 of the menstrual cycle resulted in a higher ovulation rate than with clomifene (75% versus 44%). Information regarding any potential teratogenic effects of letrozole is limited and large prospective randomised trials are required to investigate the effectiveness of aromatase inhibitors in anovulation.

Laparoscopic drilling of the ovaries

Laparoscopic drilling of the ovaries presents a further treatment option for women with anovulatory infertility associated with PCOS. It involves the creation of 4–10 perforations on the ovarian surface to a depth of 4–10 mm, using laser or unipolar coagulation. Evidence from published trials suggests comparable cumulative pregnancy rates 6–12 months after laparoscopic ovarian drilling compared with 3–6 cycles of ovulation induction with gonadotrophins.

Ovarian diathermy results in monofollicular ovulation. This means that OHSS can be avoided and the risk of multiple pregnancy reduced significantly. Laparoscopic treatment may also increase ovarian sensitivity to subsequent treatment using clomifene and gonadotrophins. Women who are slim and have high LH concentrations seem to have the most favourable prognosis.

The risks of this treatment include operative complications, especially damage to other pelvic structures that might occur with the diathermy or laser, and post-treatment adhesions. The possibility of long premature menopause due to ovarian damage is still being evaluated but, so far, in women followed up for over 10 years, there is no evidence of an increased risk. Therefore, laparoscopic ovarian drilling by laser or diathermy should be considered as an alternative to gonadotrophin treatment in women with PCOS who fail to ovulate with clomifene.

Iatrogenic problems of ovulation induction

OVARIAN HYPERSTIMULATION SYNDROME

OHSS is a potentially life-threatening effect of ovulation induction. It is rarely seen with anti-estrogens and occurs mainly following the use of gonadotrophins, especially in combination with GnRH agonists. Exposure to LH or hCG, in the form of an ovulatory trigger, luteal support or result of early pregnancy is a prerequisite for the development of OHSS.

OHSS occurs in 4% of ovulation induction cycles and is severe in 0.25–0.9%. The risks may be higher (6.6–8.4%) in IVF/ICSI cycles, where GnRH agonist is used along with gonadotrophins.

The basic pathology in OHSS is a shift of fluid from the intravascular to the extravascular space. This is caused by increased vascular permeability mediated by various agents, including LH, histamine, prostaglandins, prorenins and vascular endothelial growth factor.

The clinical symptomatology includes cystic ovarian enlargement, with accumulation of fluid in serous cavities (ascites, pleural effusion and rarely pericardial effusion). Intravascular volume depletion leads to dehydration, hypovolaemia, decreased renal perfusion, electrolyte disturbances and venous or arterial thrombosis due to the haemoconcentration.

OHSS is usually classified according to its severity (see Table 4.2).

Table 4.2 Classification of ovarian hyperstimulation syndrome (OHSS) (RCOG 2006)[5]

Grade	Symptoms
Mild	Abdominal bloating Mild abdominal pain Ovarian size usually < 8 cm[a]
Moderate	Moderate abdominal pain Nausea ± vomiting Ultrasound evidence of ascites Ovarian size usually 8–12 cm[a]
Severe	Clinical ascites (occasionally hydrothorax) Oliguria Haemoconcentration haematocrit > 45% Hypoproteinaemia Ovarian size usually > 12 cm[a]
Critical	Tense ascites or large hydrothorax Haematocrit > 55% White cell count > 25000/ml Oligo-/anuria Thromboembolism Acute respiratory distress syndrome

[a] Ovarian size may not correlate with severity of OHSS in cases of assisted reproduction because of the effect of follicular aspiration

Prevention of OHSS

Risks of OHSS can be minimised by restricting ovulation induction to centres with adequate facilities for serum E_2 and ultrasound monitoring. Use of low-dose step-up regimen, avoidance of GnRHa in ovulation induction, using pulsatile GnRH where appropriate and considering the use of metformin and laparoscopic ovarian drilling in women with PCOS can help to reduce the risk of OHSS.

If E_2 levels are excessively high or an excessive number of follicles are visualised on scan, serious consideration should be given to cycle cancellation. Withholding the ovulatory trigger of hCG can help, although a spontaneous LH surge may still trigger OHSS in the absence of GnRH agonists. Coasting (involving discontinuation of gonadotrophins in cycles with excessive response and delaying hCG administration, while continuing GnRH agonist administration), has been shown to be effective in small observational studies but lacks sufficient evidence of effect to advocate its routine use.

Treatment of OHSS

Treatment of OHSS is mainly supportive. In most cases, the condition undergoes gradual resolution over time (7 days in non-pregnant women and 10–20 days in pregnant women). There is no increase in miscarriage rates in conception cycles with OHSS.

Analgesics (paracetamol, codeine, opiates) and antiemetics can be used for the relief of discomfort and gastrointestinal symptoms. Use of anti-prostaglandins as analgesics should be avoided as they could precipitate renal failure by inhibiting renal vasodilator prostaglandins that help maintain renal blood flow. Fluid replacement to counter haemoconcentration may be oral in mild/moderate cases. Where the patient cannot tolerate oral fluids intravenous crystalloids may be used. In more severe cases, where serum albumin is less than 30 g/l or where haemoconcentration results in haemoglobin levels of more than 16 g/dl and urea levels of more than 6 mmol/l, albumin is the volume expander of choice. Infusion of 500 ml of 4.5% isotonic albumin over 2 hours can be administered quite safely in a healthy young adult but close monitoring of the haemodynamic status would be needed when larger volumes are required. Ultrasound-guided paracentesis may be required to relieve severe respiratory distress (due to abdominal distension) or to relieve pressure on the renal veins and inferior vena cava. Anti-diuretics should be avoided. Thromboembolic stockings, ambulation, correction of hypovolaemia and prophylactic anticoagulant therapy are indicated in severe cases to prevent thromboembolism.

Surgical intervention by an experienced surgeon may be required if there is torsion or rupture of the ovaries, leading to haemorrhage. As hyperstimulated ovaries are very friable and easily traumatised, surgery should be avoided unless absolutely necessary.

MULTIPLE PREGNANCY

The risks of multiple pregnancy secondary to ovulation induction vary from 7–10% for clomifene to 15–20% with gonadotrophins. More than half (52%) of higher-order multiples (triplets or more) are conceived after clomifene treatment and 33% after gonadotrophin treatment for ovulation induction.[4] A 1-year survey of triplets and higher-order pregnancies in the UK showed that 31% of triplet pregnancies were spontaneous, 34% were from the result of the different methods of ovulation induction and 35% were from assisted reproductive technology procedures.

ASSOCIATION OF OVARIAN CARCINOMA WITH OVULATION INDUCTION

A number of reports have indicated a higher than expected rate of ovarian cancer in women having drug treatment for infertility. Concerns have been raised about the exposure of the ovaries to supraphysiological levels of gonadotrophins, with multiple ovulations and trauma to the epithelial surface, resulting in the subsequent occurrence of ovarian carcinoma, when clomifene and gonadotrophins are used for ovulation induction. The extra risks posed by infertility itself make the issue difficult to evaluate. Nulliparous women with no interventions for infertility have almost double the risk of ovarian carcinoma compared with parous women. Conversely, infertile women with or without treatment who later go on to give birth have the same risk as any other parous woman without infertility. Although there is a clear association between parity and ovarian carcinoma, the available evidence does not lead to a firm link between ovulation induction agents and ovarian cancer. The risk, if it does exist, has been estimated at an annual increase of less than 1/5000. Such a risk would have to be balanced against the potential benefits of a pregnancy.

At present, it is thought that clomifene is not associated with any increased risk of ovarian cancer when used for less than 12 cycles. Until more data from large epidemiological studies become available, it would seem prudent to use gonadotrophins for the least number of cycles and at the lowest effective doses possible. Before embarking on any treatment for ovulation induction, a full discussion with the patients of the risk-benefit analysis on the current treatments available, with regard to cancer of the ovary, is advisable (Box 4.1).

KEY POINTS

- Before embarking on ovulation induction, it is essential to counsel patients regarding the risks of OHSS, multiple pregnancy, the possibility of fetal reduction and the putative risks of cancer of the ovary.
- More triplets and higher-order pregnancies follow ovulation induction rather than IVF/ICSI cycles.
- The risks of multiple pregnancy increase exponentially with every baby, for both the mother and the babies.
- There should be guidelines within every unit on reducing the risks of OHSS and multiple pregnancy, and those treatment regimens that reduce these risks.

Treatment of WHO Group I ovulatory dysfunction

DIETARY MEASURES AND PSYCHOTHERAPY

In women with weight loss or hypothalamic oligo-/amenorrhoea, weight gain resulting in a BMI of over 20 kg/m² is the most effective treatment, although this can be difficult to achieve. Women who are underweight are significantly more at risk of anaemia and preterm labour and of having babies with low birth weight or growth restriction. Treatment should therefore be deferred until dietary and psychotherapy support is provided to achieve a BMI of over 20 kg/m².

PULSATILE ADMINISTRATION OF GnRH AGONISTS

The use of pulsatile GnRH agonists is mainly indicated in women with hypogonadotrophic hypogonadism (WHO class I), where endogenous GnRH levels are very low. One example is anovulation associated with weight loss with low endogenous FSH and E_2 levels. Women who are obese and hyperandrogenic, who have polycystic ovaries with high circulating levels of LH, do not do well on this regimen. Pulsatile GnRH agonists may also be useful in the woman who is hyperprolactinaemic who cannot tolerate bromocriptine/cabergoline.

The GnRH agonist is administered subcutaneously or intravenously through a pump that must be worn round the clock. The reconstituted GnRH agonist is stable for about 3 weeks and is administered in pulses of 15–20 mg boluses for the subcutaneous dose and 5 mg boluses for the intravenous route every 60–120 minutes (usually every 90 minutes). This dose may be increased by 5 mg every week if there is no response. The patient is monitored with periodic E_2 levels and ultrasonography to detect follicular growth. Usually ovulation occurs around day 14 and the couple is advised to have intercourse around that time. The luteal phase is maintained by either continuing the pump or with hCG injections or with progestogen pessaries.

The cumulative pregnancy rates in women with hypothalamic amenorrhoea at the end of 12 cycles is around 80–90% with a 20–30% pregnancy rate/treatment cycle. The miscarriage rate is around 20% and there is no increase in congenital anomalies. The main advantage of GnRH agonist use is that the risk of multiple pregnancy is lower. The risk of OHSS is also very low and that of severe OHSS is almost nil. The problems of this regimen are more to do with the local reactions and infections at the site of needle placement or technical problems with the pump. Evidence suggests that this treatment is effective and safe in properly selected patients but it has yet to gain widespread acceptance in view of the problems of wearing the pump continuously.

GONADOTROPHIN REGIMENS

These regimens have been discussed earlier. In WHO group I ovulatory dysfunction, gonadotrophins with luteinising activity are better at inducing ovulation than pure FSH preparations.

HYPERPROLACTINAEMIA

Raised levels of prolactin interfere with the pulsatile release of GnRH from the hypothalamus. This in turn causes estrogen deficiency, anovulation and subfertility. There may be associated galactorrhoea in 30–80% of cases. Approximately 50% of women with hyperprolactinaemia show evidence of pituitary microadenoma (rarely macroadenoma), 30% have no cause detected (idiopathic). Other causes include drugs, physiological factors such as stress, renal or hepatic dysfunction and hypothyroidism where the increased thyroid-releasing hormone acts as a stimulator of prolactin secretion. About 9% of women with PCOS may have increased prolactin levels but the pathophysiology of this is not clear. Sustained hyperprolactinaemia with levels of greater than 1000 milliunits/l needs evaluation including pituitary imaging to rule out macroadenoma.

Women with macroadenoma need treatment irrespective of the severity of symptoms or the need for fertility, owing to the risk of tumour expansion. Young women with hyperprolactinaemia without evidence of a macroadenoma would also need to be treated, as they are hypoestrogenic and need estrogen to maintain skeletal integrity. In older women, bone density scanning is a useful investigation to see if hormone replacement therapy is indicated.

Treatment of hyperprolactinoma is mainly medical.

Bromocriptine

Bromocriptine is a semi-synthetic ergot alkaloid that has been in use since 1971. It is effective in shrinking 80% of macroadenomas, normalising prolactin values in 80–90% of patients and in stopping galactorrhoea and restoring ovulation in 70–80% of patients. It has a short half-life which necessitates a twice or three times daily dose. Adverse effects are commonly encountered and are mostly seen during the start of treatment. They include nausea, headache, vertigo, postural hypotension, fatigue and drowsiness. About 5% of patients need to stop treatment because of intolerable adverse effects. They can be minimised by initiating treatment with a low dose of bromocriptine (1.25 mg) at bedtime with a snack, to be gradually increased up to 2.5 mg three times a day with food over 2–3 weeks.

Cabergoline

Cabergoline is a newer dopamine agonist recently licensed for treatment of hyperprolactinaemia. It is rapidly becoming the treatment of choice for most patients, because of its many benefits over bromocriptine. These include its longer half-life, which makes its administration much simpler at 0.5–1.0 mg twice weekly. There are significantly fewer adverse effects, especially gastrointestinal. Two large randomised controlled trials have shown cabergoline to be more effective than bromocriptine in restoring normoprolactinaemia and ovulation, with fewer adverse effects.

Quinogalide

Quinogalide is another new dopamine agonist that has been found to be as effective as bromocriptine but, when compared with cabergoline, adverse effects were fewer with cabergoline. It is more expensive and is worth considering only in women resistant to bromocriptine or cabergoline.

None of these drugs has been associated with increased rates of miscarriage or congenital anomalies or any other problems with pregnancy but the current practice is to stop the drug if pregnancy occurs. This may be unnecessary with bromocriptine, particularly if there is evidence of a large prolactinoma, which may enlarge in pregnancy. Data are too few as yet with cabergoline.

Surgery

Surgery is usually indicated only in patients with non-secretory pituitary adenomas or parasellar tumours who, despite normalisation of prolactin levels and possible improvement in visual fields, do not show considerable tumour shrinkage or in patients with large macroadenomas intolerant or resistant to drug treatment. Surgery results in long-term normalisation of prolactin values only in about 50% of microadenomas and 10–15% of macroadenomas.

KEY POINTS
- Medical therapy forms the most effective and main line of treatment of hyperprolactinaemia.
- The most tried and tested dopamine agonist is bromocriptine.
- Cabergoline is rapidly becoming the drug of choice in treating hyperprolactinaemia.

Treatment options for WHO Group III ovulatory dysfunction

Egg donation is discussed in greater detail in Chapter 8 on assisted reproduction techniques but this may be the only option for women with ovarian failure. Such women should also be offered hormone replacement therapy because of the long-term problems of osteoporosis and cardiovascular disease.

Summary

In conclusion, the treatment of anovulatory infertility with currently available regimens can be very successful in many cases but is not without risk. Ovulation induction should be performed only in centres with adequate monitoring facilities and there should be clear guidelines and protocols for reducing the risks of OHSS and multiple gestation.

References

1. Rotterdam ESHRE/ASRM-sponsored PCOS consensus workshop group. Revised 2003 consensus on diagnostic criteria and long-term health risks related to polycystic ovary syndrome (PCOS). *Hum Reprod* 2004;19:41–7.
2. Lord MJ, Flight IHK, Norman RJ. Metformin in polycystic ovary syndrome: systematic review and meta-analysis. *BMJ* 2003;327,951–6.
3. Hamilton-Fairley D, Kiddy D, Watson L, Sagle M, Franks S. Low-dose gonadotrophin therapy for induction of ovulation in 100 women with polycystic ovary syndrome. *Hum Reprod* 1991;6:1095–9.
4. Levene MI, Wild J, Steer P. Higher multiple births and the modern management of infertility in Britain. The British Association of Perinatal Medicine. *Br J Obstet Gynaecol* 1992;99:507–13.
5. Royal College of Obstetricians and Gynaecologists. *The Management of Ovarian Hyperstimulation Syndrome*. Green-top Guideline No. 5. London: RCOG; 2006.

- Before embarking on ovulation induction, it is essential to counsel women regarding the risks of OHSS, multiple pregnancy and the possibility of fetal reduction and the putative risks of cancer of the ovary.
- Ovulation induction should be performed only after male and tubal factors have been ruled out. The BMI should ideally be between 20 kg/m^2 and 30 kg/m^2.
- There should be guidelines within every unit to reduce the risks of OHSS and multiple pregnancy; those treatment regimens that reduce these risks, such as low-dose gonadotrophin regimens or laparoscopic drilling of the ovaries in PCOS, should be considered.
- Pulsatile GnRH is the treatment of choice in women with hypogonadotrophic hypogonadism.
- Cabergoline is rapidly becoming the drug of choice in treating hyperprolactinaemia.

Further reading

Balen AH, Bratt DD, West C, Patel A, Jacobs HS. Cumulative conception and live birth rates after the treatment of anovulatory infertility: safety and efficacy of ovulation induction in 200 patients. *Hum Reprod* 1994;9:1563–70.

Checa MA, Requena A, Tur R, Callejo J, Espinos JJ, Fabregues F, et al. Insulin-sensitizing agents: use in pregnancy and as therapy in polycystic ovary syndrome. *Hum Reprod Update* 2005;11:375–90.

Farquhar C, Vandekerckhove P, Arnot M, Lilford R. Polycystic ovary syndrome: laparoscopic "drilling" by diathermy or laser for ovulation induction in patients with anovulatory polycystic ovarian syndrome. *Cochrane Database Syst Rev* 1998;(3).

Jenkins J, Mathur R. Ovarian hyperstimulation syndrome. PACE Review no. 98/06. In: Royal College of Obstetricians and Gynaecologists. *Personal Assessment in Continuing Education: Reviews, Questions and Answers, Volume 3*. London: RCOG Press; 2003. p. 7–9.

Webster J, Piscitelli G, Polli A, Ferrari CI, Ismail I, Scanlon MF. A comparison of cabergoline and bromocriptine in the treatment of hyperprolactinaemic amenorrhoea. *N Engl J Med* 1994;331:904–9.

5 Tubal factor infertility

Introduction

The 7–14 cm fallopian tube plays an important role in egg collection, fertilisation and embryo transport. Tubal fimbriae guide the ovulated egg into the tube. Unidirectional beating of the tubal cilia and peristaltic contractions of the muscular tubal wall transport the egg and subsequently the embryo. Secretions from the tubal epithelium facilitate fertilisation and nourish the embryo.

Tubal factor infertility includes an array of disorders affecting one or more of the above components. It may be transient or permanent and is manifested by peritubal adhesions, proximal and/or distal tubal blockage or hydrosalpinx formation (Figure 5.1). Severe impairment of tubal function can occur in the presence of a patent tube, because of damage to the inner micro-architecture.

Tubal factor infertility affects 25–35% of women who are subfertile. It is the only cause of subfertility that is potentially preventable.

Aetiology

The main causes of tubal factor infertility are infection, surgery, congenital abnormalities and endometriosis.

INFECTION

The major cause of tubal factor infertility is pelvic inflammatory disease (PID). Current methods of diagnosis and treatment of PID are unsatisfactory. Most women with tubal factor infertility give no history of past genital tract infections. Cohort studies following up women with laparoscopically confirmed PID found that the likelihood of developing tubal factor infertility after PID is related to:

- the number of episodes of PID
- severity of the episodes

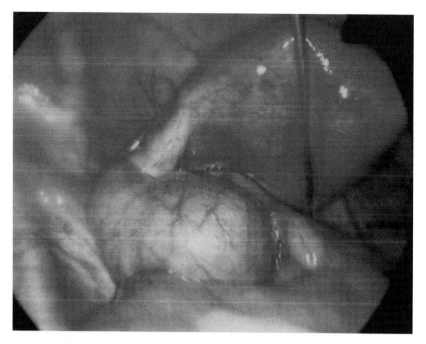

Figure 5.1 Diagnostic laparoscopy showing the uterus and right hydrosalpinx

- length of time before treatment
- age.

The risk of tubal factor infertility increases considerably with repeat infections (Table 5.1).

Most cases of PID occur after sexually transmitted infections but other organisms may play a role:

- *C. trachomatis*
- *Neisseria gonorrhoea*

Table 5.1 Increasing risk of tubal factor infertility (TFI); source Weström *et al.* 1992[1]

Episodes of PID (n)	Risk of TFI (%)
1	8
2	20
3 or more	40

- anaerobic and haemolytic streptococcus
- staphylococcus
- *Escherichia coli*
- mycoplasma
- *Clostridium perfringens*
- actinomycosis
- tuberculosis.

Of these, *C. trachomatis* is the most important. It is the most common sexually transmitted infection in the UK and is responsible for at least 60% of identifiable cases of PID. The risks of acquiring both chlamydia and PID are age related, with women less than 25 years of age at highest risk. Rates of chlamydial infection continue to rise, accelerated by its asymptomatic nature.

Anaerobic commensals are usually seen in older women or in cases of tubo-ovarian abscess. Pelvic infection secondary to actinomycosis is a rare complication of intrauterine contraceptive devices. Tuberculosis should be borne in mind if the woman is a recent immigrant from an at-risk area.

The majority of cases of PID involve ascending spread of microorganisms from the vagina and cervix to the endometrial cavity and into the fallopian tubes. Results from seroepidemiological and animal model studies show that both symptomatic and asymptomatic chlamydial infection in females can result in damage to the genital tract.

Pelvic inflammatory disease may complicate the following clinical situations or procedures:

- obstetrics:
  - vaginal delivery
  - spontaneous miscarriage
  - evacuation of retained products of conception (ERPOC)
  - medical ERPOC
  - preterm premature rupture of membranes
- gynaecology:
  - suction termination of pregnancy
  - medical termination of pregnancy
  - laparoscopy
  - hysterosalpingogram
  - hysteroscopy
  - endometrial biopsy
  - intrauterine contraceptive device insertion
  - intrauterine insemination
  - embryo transfer following IVF.

SURGERY

Lower abdominal or pelvic surgery can lead to adhesion formation. Subfertility can result due to the proximity of the operating field to the fallopian tubes. Female sterilisation involves deliberate damage to the tubes. Uterine instrumentation carries a risk of PID in the order of 5–10%.

A history of abdominal operations such as appendicectomy, bowel resection and major urological procedures may also lead to peritubal adhesions and identify women who need early tubal evaluation.

OTHER CAUSES

Congenital abnormalities affect up to 10% of females and can affect fallopian tubes. They may be associated with similar anomalies in the urinary tract.

Endometriosis accounts for 5% of female subfertility. Moderate and severe endometriosis can cause anatomic distortion of the pelvic structures. Intraluminal endometriosis is a rare cause of tubal blockage. Endometriosis is further discussed in Chapter 6.

Pathology

ACUTE INFLAMMATION

The inflammatory changes of endosalpingitis follow acute endometritis. Infection spreads to the mucosa of the fallopian tube, damaging the cilia and epithelial cells. The inflammation of interstitial salpingitis involves the whole of the tube and produces thickening of the tubal wall.

KEY POINTS
- Before undergoing uterine instrumentation, women should be offered screening for *C. trachomatis* using an appropriately sensitive technique.
- If the test is positive, women and their sexual partners should be referred for appropriate management with treatment and contact tracing.
- Prophylactic antibiotics (azithromycin 1 g orally or doxycycline 100 mg twice daily for 7 days) should be considered if screening has not been carried out.

CHRONIC INFLAMMATION

Intraluminal adhesions lead to either partial obstruction and the risk of ectopic pregnancy or complete obstruction and tubal factor infertility. Extraluminal adhesions can be secondary to salpingo-oophoritis. A pyosalpinx may form and progress to peritonitis or the inflammation may subside with development of a hydrosalpinx. Chronic PID is characterised by pelvic pain and/or dyspareunia. It is unclear whether the symptoms are secondary to the associated adhesions or due to continuing subclinical infection.

CLASSIFICATION OF TUBAL FACTOR INFERTILITY

In contrast with the accepted scoring system for pelvic endometriosis, no classification system for scoring tubal damage has gained universal acceptance. A retrospective cohort study[2] using the Hull and Rutherford classification system was able to distinguish women with tubal factor infertility into three groups:

- grade 1: filmy adhesions
- grade 2: unilateral severe damage
- grade 3: bilateral severe damage.

These grades predicted a favourable, fair or poor prognosis for live birth following tubal surgery.

Treatment

CONSERVATIVE

Figure 5.2 shows the cumulative conception rates with untreated tubal disease compared with fertile couples. The extent of tubal disease is graded from 1 (mild) to 4 (extensive). Up to 10% of the pregnancies in women with tubal factor infertility were ectopic. Overall, fecundity was much reduced in the tubal group.

MEDICAL

Tubal infection may persist despite repeated courses of antibiotics, while the role of antibiotic therapy in cases of tubal factor infertility secondary to PID is unproven.

Evidence suggests that tubal flushing with an oil-soluble contrast media will increase pregnancy rates compared with no intervention.

Women with tuberculosis require chemotherapy but this will not reverse the damage present. After treatment, increased ectopic and miscarriage rates are reported on a background of decreased conception.

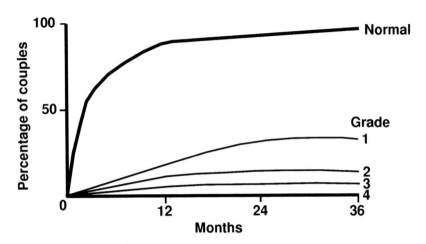

Figure 5.2   Cumulative conception rates related to disease grading, compared with normal (adapted from Wu and Gocial 1988)[2]

SURGERY

Surgery offers the best results when carried out on properly selected women. It has an important complementary role to IVF in the management of patients with tubal factor infertility. Counselling is complex and a number of factors should be taken into account before a decision is made to embark on surgery (Table 5.2).

Unlike IVF, the effect of surgery is not limited to one or more episodes of treatment. However, this needs to be weighed against an increased risk of an ectopic pregnancy.

Surgical options

PROXIMAL TUBAL OBSTRUCTION

Proximal tubal obstruction may occur in either the intramural segment or uterotubal junction. It accounts for 10–25% of tubal factor infertility. Causes include:

- obliterative fibrosis
- salpingitis isthmica nodosa
- congenital abnormalities
- polyps
- intramucosal endometriosis
- chronic inflammation.

Table 5.2	Factors to be taken into account prior to embarking on surgery
Factor	Considerations for treatment
Female age	Fecundity dramatically decreases after 40 years of age
Cause of tubal disease	In cases of tubal factor infertility due to tuberculosis, for example, medical management followed by IVF would be most appropriate
Extent of tubal disease	In general, the more severe the tubal disease, the lower the pregnancy rate and the higher the ectopic rate when treated by surgery
Previous surgery	A woman with a history of an ectopic pregnancy has a risk (approximately 15%) of recurrence
Presence of other infertility factors	These may identify those who would most benefit from assisted reproduction
Surgical experience and appropriate facilities	Tubal surgery should only be carried out by operators and assistants who have appropriate facilities and sufficient patient throughput to maintain experience
Financial	The cost of privately funded treatment may be beyond the couple's means

Therapeutic approaches include tubal cannulation, tubocornual anastomosis and IVF. However, in up to 40% of women proximal tubal obstruction is the result of tubal spasm or transient occlusion by mucous plugs.

SELECTIVE SALPINGOGRAPHY WITH TUBAL CANNULATION

Diagnostic selective salpingography differentiates true proximal tubal obstruction from blocks due to spasm or plugs and can delineate the exact site(s) of occlusion. Recognised contraindications include pregnancy, active pelvic infection and allergy to the contrast media.

A preliminary HSG is undertaken (Figure 5.3) and then salpingography performed by advancing a curved catheter into the tubal ostium. The cannula is abutted against the intrauterine ostia and radio-opaque dye is injected into the fallopian tube.

Tubal cannulation uses catheters, guidewires or balloon systems to attempt recanalisation (Figure 5.4). The approach is either sonographic, fluoroscopic or hysteroscopic. While the majority of occlusions can be overcome, reocclusion can occur. Complications include tubal perforation, infection, minor bleeding, vasovagal reactions and potential cancer risks associated with radiation exposure.

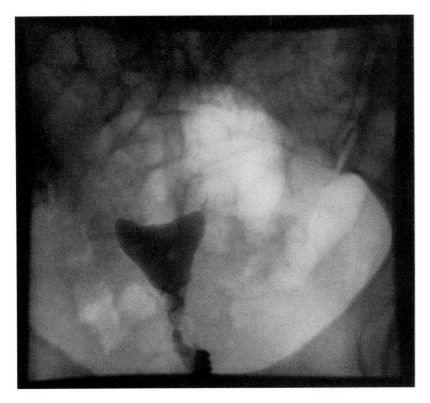

Figure 5.3　Hysterosalpingogram showing bilateral proximal tubal obstruction

The procedure takes approximately 30 minutes and offers simultaneous outpatient diagnosis and treatment (Figure 5.5). The different methods have not been compared, so it is not possible to recommend one over another. They are only available in specialist centres and are more likely to benefit those with mucous plugs and synechiae than occlusive wall disease. Evidence suggests that selective salpingography and tubal catheterisation/hysteroscopic transcervical tubal cannulation can achieve pregnancy rates of 9–57%. No randomised trials or observational studies have compared tubal catheterisation with conservative management. The measurement of tubal perfusion pressures may play a prognostic role in the future.

For women with proximal tubal disease, selective salpingography plus tubal catheterisation or hysteroscopic tubal cannulation may be treatment options because they improve the chances of pregnancy.

Surgical management also includes tubocornual anastomosis. This carries a risk of pregnancy-related uterine rupture if the procedure breaches the myometrium. The microsurgical approach produces higher

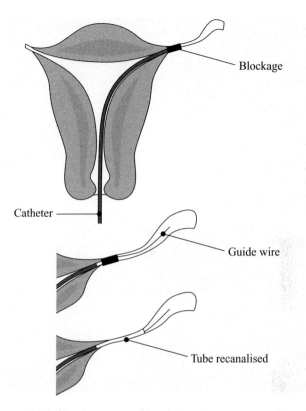

Catheter

Blockage

Guide wire

Tube recanalised

Figure 5.4   Tubal catheterisation

pregnancy rates. There are no randomised controlled trials or controlled studies that compare proximal tubal obstruction surgery with no treatment, tubal catheterisation or IVF.

DISTAL TUBAL OBSTRUCTION

Distal tubal obstruction accounts for 85% of all cases of tubal factor infertility and is caused by PID, adhesions from previous surgery and endometriosis. Therapeutic approaches include surgery and IVF.

Non-randomised studies report higher pregnancy rates in women who underwent surgery compared with those who did not. Outcome was closely linked to the severity of tubal damage, with surgery being most effective in mild disease. Pregnancy rates after tubal surgery were comparable to those following IVF in women with mild adhesions or distal blockage.

Evidence suggests the following:

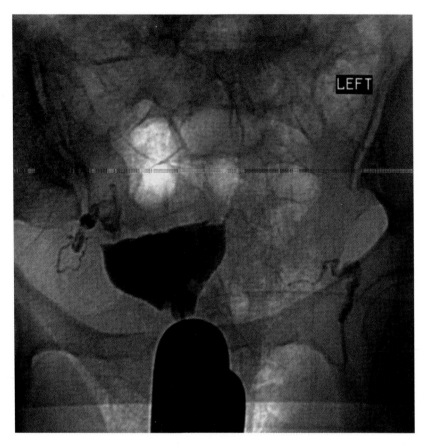

Figure 5.5   Bilateral tubal patency following tubal catheterisation

- no difference in pregnancy rates between CO_2 laser and diathermy for adhesiolysis and salpingostomy
- no difference using an operating microscope versus magnifying lenses
- no difference between laparoscopic and microsurgical adhesiolysis techniques.

Reversal of sterilisation

Approximately 5% of women will regret being sterilised and 1% will request reversal. The most common reason is a new relationship. Careful preoperative counselling can decrease but not eliminate the number of such requests.

The following factors should be taken into account when deciding whether a woman is suitable for reversal of sterilisation:

- commitment and stability of relationship: GP or social work evaluation
- fitness for surgery
- female age: women aged 35 years or less have higher pregnancy rates
- presence of coexisting tubal pathology: IVF may be more appropriate
- presence of other infertility factors: IVF may be more appropriate
- type of sterilisation technique used: clips and Silastic® rings destroy less tube than electrocauterisation
- surgical experience and appropriate facilities: success rates are related to the experience of the surgeon and high pregnancy rates can be achieved using a microsurgical approach.

Confirmation of ovulation and semen analysis is mandatory prior to undertaking reversal of sterilisation.

Isthmic-isthmic anastomosis is the most successful. Results are poorer when the ampulla is damaged or when there is disparity in the luminal diameter of the two joined segments.

Even in women over 40 years of age, reversal can achieve high intrauterine pregnancy rates, while IVF success rates tend to be poor. Reported pregnancy rates range from 31–90%.

No randomised controlled trials comparing reversal of sterilisation and IVF exist. Compared with IVF, reversal surgery allows for repeated attempts at conception. It also carries no risk of ovarian hyperstimulation and lower risks of multiple pregnancy and miscarriage. These, however, must be balanced against the risks of major abdominal surgery and an increased ectopic rate.

In general, tubal factor infertility due to female sterilisation should be treated by tubal reanastomosis, not by IVF.

KEY POINTS
- Surgery offers acceptable results only when carried out in properly selected women.
- If effective, it enables couples to conceive naturally without further intervention.
- Compared with IVF, tubal surgery carries no risk of ovarian hyperstimulation and a lower risk of both multiple pregnancy and miscarriage.
- Ectopic pregnancy is a possible outcome with all surgical techniques.
- Most cases of infertility due to female sterilisation should be treated by tubal reanastomosis.

What if surgery fails?

There is insufficient evidence to support the routine practice of hydrotubation or second-look laparoscopy after tubal surgery. Most studies considering pregnancy following surgery for proximal and distal tubal disease and tubal reanastomosis report that the majority of pregnancies occur in the first year. It is reasonable to discuss IVF with a couple that are not pregnant 12–18 months after tubal surgery.

In vitro fertilisation

IVF was first introduced to overcome tubal infertility. It should be considered first-line treatment for moderate, severe and bipolar tubal disease. However, as data from a systematic review show lower live birth rates in the presence of hydrosalpinges, laparoscopic salpingectomy should be considered prior to IVF.

Women with hydrosalpinges should be offered salpingectomy, preferably by laparoscopy, before IVF treatment because this improves the chance of a live birth.

From 1998–1999, women with tubal factor infertility underwent 10 923 cycles of IVF (31% of the total). The live birth rate was 16% compared with 17% overall. Current figures are not available.

IVF or surgery?

When deciding on treatment for a couple with tubal factor infertility, patient selection and number of IVF cycles available are the most important factors. By reserving surgery for women with proximal tubal obstruction, low-grade disease and reversal of clip sterilisation, the number of operations can be reduced, repeated attempts at conception are allowed and good live birth rates can be achieved.

One life table analysis reported that over 70% of women with tubal factor infertility will have a live birth within four cycles of IVF treatment. This must be balanced, however, against the risks of ovarian hyperstimulation, multiple pregnancies and the fact that, at present, the majority of British women have fewer cycles of IVF.

Both surgery and IVF should be discussed without bias, bearing in mind that no randomised controlled comparison of the two exists. Prognosis should be individualised, taking into account local experience and outcomes. In particular, women should be informed that the chance of a live birth declines with age, especially for those aged 40 years and over.

Prevention

Tubal factor infertility is the only preventable cause of infertility. Preventative measures include the following:

- good technique during pelvic surgery, including the use of unpowdered gloves, minimal tissue handling, sharp dissection, irrigation and meticulous haemostasis.
- absorbable adhesion barriers significantly decrease the incidence, extent and severity of postoperative adhesions. However, they are costly and there is no evidence of their effect on pregnancy rates.
- *C. trachomatis* screening or antibiotic prophylaxis if undertaking uterine instrumentation.
- opportunistic screening for *C. trachomatis* of all sexually active women under the age of 25 years and those over 25 years if they have a new sexual partner or two or more partners in the past 12 months.

Worldwide, there has been an increase in the prevalence of chlamydial infection. Programmes to decrease the incidence of genital chlamydial infection have not been widely implemented except in Sweden, where screening, contact tracing and free treatment have been in place since the 1980s. Declining rates of chlamydial infection, PID and ectopic pregnancy have been attributed to these policies. Randomised data support the benefit of targeted screening, with a halving of PID rates at 1 year.

A large UK pilot study found chlamydial infection to be present in 11% of sexually active women under 20 years. In response, the Department of Health has started a national screening programme in selected areas in England targeting women (and to a lesser extent men) less than 25 years of age.

References

1. Westrom L, Joesoef R, Reynolds G, Hagdu A, Thompson SE. Pelvic inflammatory disease and infertility: a cohort study of 1844 women with laparoscopically verified disease and 657 control women with normal laparoscopic results. *Sex Transm Dis* 1992;19:185–92.
2. Wu CH, Gocial B. A pelvic scoring system for infertility surgery. *Int J Fertil* 1988;33:341–6.
3. Akande VA, Cahill DJ, Wardle PG, Rutherford AJ, Jenkins M. The predictive value of "Hull & Rutherford" classification for tubal damage. *BJOG* 2004;111:1236–41.

Further reading

Khalaf Y. Tubal subfertility. *BMJ* 2003;327:610–13.
National Collaborating Centre for Women's and Children's Health. *Fertility: Assessment and Treatment for People with Fertility Problems*. London: RCOG Press; 2004.

6 Infertility and endometriosis

Introduction

Endometriosis, defined as the presence of viable endometrial tissue outside the uterine cavity, is a common condition affecting 2–3% of women of reproductive age. Many aspects of the pathogenesis of endometriosis are unknown and its aetiology appears to be multifactorial. Today, a composite theory of retrograde menstruation with implantation of endometrial fragments, in conjunction with peritoneal factors that stimulate cell growth, is the most widely accepted explanation. The sequelae of endometriosis include chronic pelvic pain, severe dysmenorrhoea and infertility. The presence and severity of symptoms do not correspond directly with the extent of visible disease.

The association with infertility is unclear. Endometriosis is diagnosed in 10–20% of women investigated for infertility compared with 1–5% of women undergoing sterilisation. Despite intense research over the past 50 years, the pathophysiological mechanisms of endometriosis and endometriosis-associated reproductive failure remain incompletely understood. Reduced fecundity in women with moderate and severe endometriosis can be explained by anatomical alterations associated with pelvic adhesions (Figure 6.1). The effects of minimal and mild endometriosis on fertility are less straightforward, although the monthly fecundity rate in these women is lower than that of the general population (Figure 6.2).

The lack of good quality, prospective, controlled studies and inconsistencies in staging make it difficult to be certain that the mere presence of endometriosis affects fertility. It is possible that an underlying defect, possibly of immunological origin, may be responsible for both endometriosis as well as infertility in women with endometriosis.

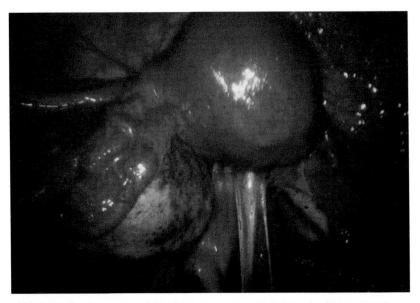

Figure 6.1   Left ovarian endometrioma and peritoneal deposits (reproduced with permission from *An Atlas of Endometriosis*, by RW Shaw, Parthenon Publishing Group)

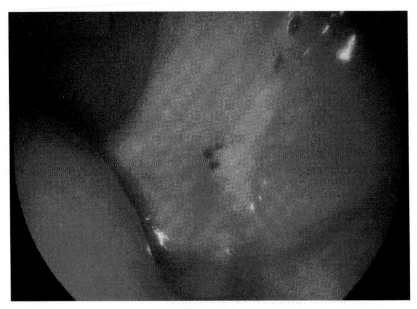

Figure 6.2   Mild endometriosis (reproduced with permission from *An Atlas of Endometriosis*, by RW Shaw, Parthenon Publishing Group)

Mechanisms by which minimal and mild endometriosis may impair fertility

DEFECTIVE FOLLICULOGENESIS

It has been suggested that, in women with endometriosis, ovulation may be disturbed by an abnormality of the follicular growth rate and total growth period. Alternatively, altered intra-ovarian mechanisms might be responsible for abnormal follicular recruitment, growth and selection. No significant differences in terms of endocrinology, folliculogenesis, endogenous LH surge and endometrial thickness have been demonstrated in women with or without endometriosis.

DISORDERS OF OVULATION

Luteinised unruptured follicle syndrome refers to a condition where, following normal follicular growth and estrogen secretion, a follicle fails to rupture and release the oocyte. This does not prevent subsequent luteinisation of the granulosa cells. Laparoscopic examination and serial ultrasound scans during the luteal phase have failed to confirm whether this occurs more often in women with endometriosis. It has also been suggested that anovulation is more common in infertile women with endometriosis but this has never been confirmed.

HYPERPROLACTINAEMIA

Hyperprolactinaemia has been reported in 11–36% of women with mild endometriosis. It has been suggested that women with endometriosis demonstrate a significant increase in the prolactin response to thyroid-releasing hormone (TRH). However, this increase was found to be confined to women with severe endometriosis. The mechanism by which women with endometriosis exhibit significant prolactinaemia following an LHRH/TRH test is unclear. The administration of bromocriptine as a therapeutic measure has been tried but available data suggest that it is ineffective.

LUTEAL PHASE DEFICIENCY

The diagnosis of luteal phase deficiency is based upon either:

- the duration of the luteal phase
- an aberrant basal body temperature chart and endometrial biopsy
- a low level of progesterone production.

It was initially suggested that women with endometriosis demonstrated decreased progesterone production during the luteal phase. However, studies based on single and multiple progesterone estimations have shown that luteal progesterone production in such women is normal. It is therefore reasonable to conclude that a luteal phase defect is not the mechanism by which the majority of women with endometriosis are rendered infertile.

IMPAIRED IMPLANTATION

Mounting evidence suggests that disorders of endometrial function may contribute to the decreased fecundity observed in women with endometriosis. Reduced endometrial expression of the a and b integrins (a cell adhesion molecule) during the time of implantation has been described in some women with endometriosis. Very low levels of an enzyme involved in the synthesis of the endometrial ligand for L-section (a protein that coats the trophoblast on the surface of the blastocyst) have been observed in infertile women with endometriosis.[1] These data lend credence to the hypothesis that functional disorders of the endometrium may both predispose to the development of endometriosis and impair implantation mechanisms in affected women.

AUTOIMMUNITY

It has been suggested that sensitisation to endometrial antigens could occur as part of the inflammatory response to the retrograde menstrual debris: the resultant autoantibodies could thus interfere with the process of fertilisation and possibly implantation. An increase in the number of T cells, B cells and the ratio of CD4/CD8 lymphocytes in women with endometriosis in both peritoneal fluid and peripheral blood has also been reported. The methods used in many of these studies were non-specific and some of the earlier findings were later refuted by further studies.

PERITONEAL ENVIRONMENT

Endometriosis can now be regarded as a local inflammatory process in the pelvis. The local environment of peritoneal fluid surrounding the endometrial implant is immunologically dynamic and links the reproductive and immune systems. The fallopian tubes and ovaries are bathed in peritoneal fluid. Spermatozoa are exposed to peritoneal fluid factors in the fallopian tube before and during fertilisation, as are oocytes and embryos.

The volume of peritoneal fluid in women with endometriosis may be increased but this appears to be of little clinical importance and correlates poorly with infertility. However, some components of peritoneal fluid could have a negative effect on the reproductive environment. This may be associated with the increased concentration of macrophages that exist in the presence of endometriosis. It is becoming evident that cytokines, released by macrophages, play an important role in reproduction at various levels, including gamete function, fertilisation and embryo development, implantation and post-implantation survival of the conceptus. Overall, there appears to be enough evidence to suggest that the peritoneal environment in women with endometriosis is relatively hostile to the process of conception.

KEY POINTS
- Endometriosis is more frequently diagnosed among infertile women than in fertile women.
- Owing to the lack of controlled studies and of agreement on the consistency of staging, it is uncertain whether the presence of endometriosis reduces fertility.
- In advanced endometriosis adhesion formation and tubal damage can directly affect fertility.

The majority of studies are inconclusive regarding the possible mechanisms by which minimal and mild endometriosis may impair fertility.

Treatment of endometriosis and reproductive outcome

The management of endometriosis remains contentious. There are many reports in the literature on therapeutic options for endometriosis, but data from well-designed studies supporting the effectiveness of these interventions are not always available. This is particularly true for women with minimal and mild disease, in whom no clear causal association can be defined. The options for treatment of endometriosis-associated infertility include:

- no treatment (expectant management)
- medical treatment with or without surgery
- surgical treatment by laparoscopy or laparotomy.

Existing studies have a number of methodological problems. These include clinical heterogeneity in terms of disease stage and the presence of comorbidity, small sample sizes and variable duration of follow-up.

MEDICAL TREATMENT

Pharmacological agents used for the medical treatment of endometriosis include:

- continuous combined oral contraceptive preparations
- progestogens
- danazol
- gestrinone
- aromatase inhibitors
- GnRH-agonists.

In the treatment of endometriosis-associated infertility, the best quality data available demonstrate no benefit from ovulation suppression when compared to placebo or no treatment, whatever the stage of the disease. Three systematic reviews, all using slightly different methodologies, have consistently shown that there is no significant difference in crude pregnancy rates between medical treatment and no treatment in endometriosis. In the cohort studies included in the one meta-analysis,[2] there was no evidence to suggest that medical treatment of endometriosis improved fertility. Therefore, medical treatment causing ovulation suppression is not appropriate for endometriosis-related infertility. Larger trials do not appear to be warranted on the basis of available data.

SURGICAL TREATMENT

In moderate and severe endometriosis, comparisons of surgical treatments with non-surgical alternatives show that surgery is generally superior, in terms of pregnancy rates. There is, however, no evidence of a difference between laparoscopic and open (laparotomy) approaches.

It is less clear whether surgery is superior to no treatment in minimal and mild disease. Laparotomy for the treatment of minimal or mild disease would generally be regarded as inappropriate. Data from nine studies comparing laparoscopic surgery with no treatment in minimal and mild endometriosis showed an increased relative risk of pregnancy of 1.6 (95% CI 1.4–1.8), in favour of laparoscopic resection or ablation. These studies included a large well-designed randomised trial by Marcoux et al.[3] where 341 infertile women with minimal and mild endometriosis were randomised to either diagnostic laparoscopy alone or laparoscopy along with surgical treatment of the endometriosis and lysis of adhesions. Its results suggested that laparoscopic surgery increased the cumulative probability of a pregnancy by 73% in the first 36 weeks after the procedure. This suggests a benefit from resection or ablation of endometriosis to one in eight women with minimal or mild disease undergoing such a procedure. The women in this trial were not blinded to their treatment; 14% of women had lysis of adhesions as well as destruction of endometriosis and a small number also underwent co-interventions such as ovulation induction, IVF/IUI, progestogens, cyst excision and contraception.

In an Italian trial,[4] 20% of treated women and 22% of those untreated had a successful outcome (conceived within 1 year and had a live birth). When the results of Canadian and Italian studies are combined, the overall absolute difference is 8.6% in favour of therapy. The number needed to treat is 12. Thus, for every 12 women with stage I–II endometriosis treated with ablation/resection of endometriosis, there will be one additional pregnancy. There is no evidence that the outcome is affected by the method of ablation, by electrosurgery or laser delivery systems. It is clear, however, that there is a need for further controlled prospective studies that present their results for different stages of endometriosis using comparable classification systems.

ADJUVANT TREATMENT

Available evidence suggests that in the management of endometriosis-associated infertility, the addition of postoperative medical treatment does not improve pregnancy rates compared to surgery alone. This is true whether the surgery involves either laparoscopy or laparotomy. Thus, it seems clear that medical treatment, whether alone or after surgery, has no role in the management of endometriosis-associated infertility.

There is still the possibility that presurgical medical treatment could be a beneficial adjunct. The theoretical advantages of medical treatment before surgery are reduced inflammation and vascularisation and shrinkage of implants. However, the quality of evidence supporting the use of medical treatment before conservative surgery for endometriosis is poor and no recommendations can be made based on the results of the published studies.

KEY POINTS
- Medical treatment has no role in the management of endometriosis-associated infertility.
- Surgery is generally superior to non-surgical alternatives in moderate and severe endometriosis.
- Subfertile women also benefit from surgical ablation of minimal and mild endometriosis.

Assisted reproduction in endometriosis-related infertility

Pelvic endometriosis refractory to medical or surgical therapy currently accounts for between 7% and 35% of women undergoing IVF procedures. All stages of endometriosis have increasingly been viewed as suitable indications for assisted reproduction treatment. However, it is not known whether IVF or gamete intrafallopian transfer (GIFT) is better than medical or surgical treatment for endometriosis associated infertility. Following the advent of assisted reproduction, more women with endometriosis who fail to conceive with conventional therapy have been treated with one or the other of these techniques. The timing of assisted reproduction is dependent upon the severity of the disease and any previous therapy, as well as other factors, such as female age and duration of infertility.

There are no direct comparisons of relevance but some evidence suggests that IVF or GIFT may be better than conventional treatment for women with endometriosis, whatever the stage of disease (Table 6.1). As far as the success of IVF or GIFT treatment is concerned, large national registers have repeatedly reported similar pregnancy rates for women with endometriosis in comparison with other categories. The presence or the degree of endometriosis does not appear to affect the fertilisation or embryo cleavage rates and, more particularly the live birth rates following treatment. However, one study demonstrated the benefits of prolonged down-regulation with GnRHa before initiation of IVF-embryo transfer in women with endometriosis.[5]

Table 6.1   Use of assisted reproduction in endometriosis-related infertility

Severity of endometriosis	Treatment
Minimal or mild	IVF or GIFT treatment after more than 2 years of surgical or expectant management IUI with ovarian hyperstimulation may be an effective alternative to IVF (used for at least three cycles)
Moderate or severe	IVF should be considered 1 year after unsuccessful surgery IVF may be considered in preference to surgery depending on the clinical situation
Severe, with mechanical blockage and where surgical therapy is inappropriate	IVF should be expedited

Evidence on the use of IUI in the treatment of endometriosis-associated infertility suggests that superovulation in conjunction with IUI is more effective than no treatment in women with minimal or mild disease.

KEY POINTS

- The timing of assisted reproduction is dependent on the severity of the disease and any previous therapy, as well as other factors, such as female age and duration of infertility.
- IVF or GIFT may be better than conventional treatment for women with endometriosis, whatever the stage of disease.
- In cases of moderate and severe endometriosis, assisted reproductive techniques should be considered, as an alternative to or following unsuccessful surgery.
- In cases of minimal or mild disease IVF or IUI with ovarian stimulation may be considered after more than two years of surgical or expectant management.

Summary

The nature of the relationship between endometriosis and infertility remains unresolved. It is unclear whether endometriosis causes infertility or whether there is an underlying defect that causes both infertility and endometriosis. Clinical decisions in the management of infertility associated with endometriosis are difficult because of the paucity of randomised controlled trials.

There seems to be enough evidence to suggest that drugs suppressing ovulation are of no benefit in infertile women with endometriosis and their use only delays the likelihood of a spontaneous pregnancy. For infertile women with suspected stage I–II endometriosis, a decision must be made whether to perform laparoscopic ablation before offering either conventional fertility treatments or assisted reproduction. Factors such as the woman's age, duration of infertility, family history and pelvic pain must be taken into consideration.

References

1. Kao LC, Germeyer A, Tulac S, Lobo S, Yang JP, Taylor RN, *et al*. Expression profiling of endometrium from women with endometriosis reveals candidate genes for disease-based implantation failure and infertility. *Endocrinology* 2003;144:2870–81.

2. Adamson GD, Pasta DJ. Surgical treatment of endometriosis-associated infertility: meta-analysis compared with survival analysis. *Am J Obstet Gynecol* 1994;171:1488–504.
3. Marcoux S, Maheux R, Berube S. Laparoscopic surgery in infertile women with minimal or mild endometriosis. *N Engl J Med* 1997;337:217–22.
4. Parazzini F. Ablation of lesions or no treatment in minimal–mild endometriosis in infertile women: a randomized trial. Gruppo Italiano per lo Studio dell'Endometriosi. *Hum Reprod* 1999;14:1332–4.
5. Surrey ES, Silverberg KM, Surrey MW, Schoolcraft WB. Effect of prolonged gonadotropin-releasing hormone analogue treatment on preclinical abortions in patients with severe endometriosis undergoing in vitro fertilization-embryo transfer. *Fertil Steril* 2002;78:699–704.

Further reading

Practice Committee of the American Society for Reproductive Medicine. Endometriosis and infertility. *Fertil Steril* 2004;82:S40–5.

7 Unexplained infertility

Introduction

Infertility is described as unexplained where routine investigations such as semen analysis, tubal patency and assessment of ovulation yield normal results. Intrinsic differences within populations and variations in investigation protocols have led to a wide range in the reported prevalence of unexplained infertility, ranging between 5.8% and 58.0%, although most clinics report a figure of 20–30%. The clinical approach to unexplained infertility has undergone a major shift in emphasis. In the past, the aim was to identify potential biological causes for the condition in the hope of devising appropriate therapy. In the absence of a recognised cause, a number of treatments have been used without any scientific proof of effectiveness. Availability of assisted reproduction, reliance on evidence based treatments and awareness of the need to limit adverse effects have redefined our management of unexplained infertility. This chapter considers some of the putative causes of unexplained infertility before assessing the effectiveness of common strategies of investigation and treatment in the light of available evidence.[1]

Possible causes of unexplained infertility

Failure of routine tests to detect any obvious causes has led clinicians to speculate about numerous subtle factors that may be responsible for unexplained infertility. Although many of these remain of interest to researchers, their practical relevance has been diminished by the growing role of assisted reproduction.

LUTEAL-PHASE DEFICIENCY

Luteal-phase deficiency as a cause of unexplained infertility remains a controversial topic. Presumed to be due to defects in folliculogenesis and luteal function, potential mechanisms include abnormalities of gonadotrophin secretion, endometrial steroid receptor function and luteal rescue mechanisms. While delays in histological maturation of the endometrium have been cited as proof of the existence of this condition, its effect on fertility is unclear. Lack of consensus about both diagnosis and treatment of this condition have challenged its clinical relevance in recent years.

LUTEINISED UNRUPTURED FOLLICLE SYNDROME

Failure of the leading follicle to rupture in the presence of biochemical evidence of ovulation has been linked to unexplained infertility. Following the LH peak, serial ultrasound scans have identified failure of the dominant follicle to shrink in a group of women with low serum progesterone levels. Its clinical usefulness is compromised by the lack of uniformity of ultrasonic criteria defining this syndrome.

HYPERPROLACTINAEMIA

The role of prolactin in ovulatory disorders remains uncertain. High levels of prolactin may be associated with deficient luteal function. Both transient elevations of prolactin in the luteal phase and absence of the midcycle elevation of prolactin have been demonstrated in women with unexplained infertility. However, prolactin-lowering agents such as bromocriptine have been ineffective in treating women with unexplained infertility.

Although it is difficult to identify specific hormonal derangements in women with unexplained infertility, intensive monitoring can reveal subtle abnormalities suggestive of diminished ovarian reserve. Most workers now accept the limitations of screening for mild ovarian dysfunction. Evidence linking other subtle endocrine abnormalities to unexplained infertility is tenuous and there is little justification for empirical hormonal treatment.

ENDOMETRIOSIS

Mild endometriosis without any distortion of pelvic anatomy has traditionally been treated in the same way as unexplained infertility. The association between endometriosis and infertility and treatment of mild endometriosis are discussed in Chapter 6.

SUBCLINICAL PREGNANCY LOSS

Once considered to be an important factor in unexplained infertility, the prevalence of this condition has been shown to be no different from that in the general population.

ANATOMICAL ABNORMALITIES

Tubocornual polyps and other subtle anatomical aberrations are of little relevance in the causation of unexplained infertility and their treatment seems to have minimal effect.

OCCULT INFECTION

Impaired tubal function due to previous infection with *Chlamydia trachomatis* has been cited as a possible aetiology for unexplained infertility. Although chlamydia infection is clearly important in the context of tubal disease, the role of infection in the genesis of unexplained infertility is unproven. Currently, there is no evidence to support the empirical use of antibiotics in unexplained infertility.

SPERM DYSFUNCTION

Conventional semen analysis represents a crude method of assessing male fertility, particularly as it cannot evaluate the functional capacity of spermatozoa. Some cases of unexplained infertility could be associated with subtle disorders of sperm function as well as sperm–mucus and sperm–oocyte interaction, which can only be exposed by IVF. Cellular defects of sperm may relate to the generation of abnormal amounts of free oxygen radicals, which could affect the stability of the sperm membrane. Such sperm may be functionally incompetent despite possessing normal laboratory parameters. Though sophisticated tests of sperm function remain useful research tools, access to assisted reproduction and the current role of IVF as a test of gamete function limit their role in current management of unexplained infertility.

IMMUNOLOGICAL CAUSES

Serological tests have identified the presence of anti-sperm antibodies capable of inhibiting fertilisation, although a clear link between the presence of these antibodies and unexplained infertility has yet to be established. Antiphospholipid antibodies, including antibodies to any one of five to seven phospholipid antigens, have been linked with infertility. As assays for antiphospholipid antibodies other than anticardiolipin are not standardised, this is a difficult association to prove.

PSYCHOLOGICAL FACTORS

Although infertility is undoubtedly stressful, proof of a direct correlation between objectively defined stress levels and unexplained infertility is unavailable. Conversely, no controlled studies exist that show a link between reduction of stress and enhanced fertility in this group.

Diagnosis

Investigation of the infertile couple is discussed in Chapter 2. Complete evaluation of the pelvis requires a diagnostic laparoscopy with dye transit. However, because of logistic problems and concern about risks of surgery, it is considered acceptable to perform HSG in women without a history of high risk factors for tubal infertility. Where basic tests for ovulation, semen parameters and tubal patency are all normal and the pelvis is unremarkable, unexplained infertility is the diagnosis of exclusion. Available evidence does not support routine use of tests such as endometrial biopsy, serial progesterone levels and ovarian scans in an attempt to diagnose luteal phase deficiency. Sperm function tests and tests for anti-sperm antibodies are also not recommended. Much debate still surrounds the use of the postcoital test. It has been found to be useful in predicting spontaneous conception in couples with a short duration of infertility (less than 3 years) where female causes of infertility have been excluded. A systematic review of observational studies has failed to confirm the predictive power of this test while a randomised trial on 444 women has failed to demonstrate any advantages of routine postcoital testing in terms of cumulative pregnancy rates. Intervention rates were found to be higher in women subjected to the investigation.

Other investigations that have yet to be shown to be clinically useful include screening for antiphospholipid antibodies, hysteroscopy and ultrasound of the endometrium.

Management

From the outset, it must be appreciated that the management of unexplained infertility has certain unique features. Firstly, in the absence of a certain diagnosis, any form of treatment is, by nature, speculative. Secondly, treatment, including relatively invasive assisted reproduction techniques offer fairly modest live-birth rates. Thirdly, the very real chance of a spontaneous pregnancy must be taken into account when treatment is considered. This treatment independent pregnancy rate is strongly affected by the duration of infertility (Figure 7.1). A period of 3 years of unexplained infertility is generally accepted as the minimum duration before considering active intervention. In couples who have been trying for less than 3 years, the likelihood of spontaneous pregnancy over the next 2 years is 46% as opposed to 28% in those with a longer duration of infertility.[2] In addition, two other factors – female age

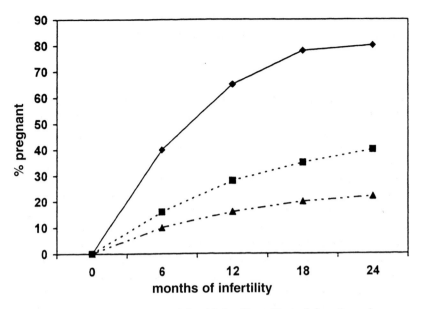

Figure 7.1 Prognosis in unexplained infertility: effect of duration of infertility; − - ▲ - − = 1 year; -■- = 3–5 years; −− = over 5 years

and previous pregnancy – have a major effect on spontaneous conception rates as well as treatment outcome (see Table 1.3, Chapter 1).

A number of models for estimating the chance of conception in unexplained infertility have been devised. In women under 35 years of age, conservative treatment for up to 3 years should be considered, since spontaneous conception rates only start to decline significantly after this period. Successful communication with the couple is vital and the importance of detailed discussion and written information sheets cannot be overstated. Many couples feel frustrated by the apparent refusal to accede to their request for early treatment and need careful counselling.

Once the expectant role is abandoned, it is important to identify the treatment of choice and formulate a clear plan of future management. When a number of options are available it may be appropriate to start with one that is least invasive. Management should be evidence based, consistent with the wishes of the couple and sensitive to financial constraints.

The effectiveness of some of the commonly used forms of treatment is discussed below.

EMPIRICAL CLOMIFENE

Clomifene citrate has been shown to increase the number of follicles produced per cycle, thus increasing the odds of a fertilised embryo reaching the uterine cavity. Its use in unexplained infertility is still open to debate. A meta-analysis has demonstrated a statistically significant benefit following the use of clomifene in unexplained infertility.[3] The combined odds ratio for clinical pregnancy/woman was 2.37 (CI 1.43–3.94). The small sample size of the individual trials included in this review inevitably means that the present conclusions are likely to be affected by the outcome of future larger studies. Traditionally, clomifene has been viewed as a relatively innocuous drug and its empirical use preferred by many to the more invasive assisted reproduction techniques. Concerns about clomifene-induced multiple pregnancy and inability to rule out a potential link with ovarian cancer underline the need to weigh the risk–benefit ratio carefully. The approach to the use of clomifene in unexplained infertility differs from that in anovulatory women. A starting dose of 50 mg is used and a day 12 ultrasound scan performed to assess ovarian follicular response. If the ovarian response is very brisk, which occurs in as many as 15% of cases, the dose should be cut down to 25 mg. The aim is to achieve no more than two preovulatory follicles over 17 mm.

INTRAUTERINE INSEMINATION WITH OR WITHOUT SUPEROVULATION

Superovulation and IUI has been a recognised treatment for unexplained infertility for a number of years. Though this approach is less invasive than IVF, significant risks of ovarian stimulation and multiple pregnancy remain. Current evidence regarding this treatment comes from a meta-analysis of eight randomised controlled trials showing that gonadotrophins plus IUI led to higher pregnancy rates compared to gonadotrophins plus timed intercourse (OR 2.37, 95% CI 1.43–3.90).[4] A second analysis of 22 trials indicates that the independent OR for pregnancy associated with IUI 2.82 (95% CI 2.18–3.66).

IUI in natural (unstimulated) cycles as well as in combination with superovulation has been used to treat unexplained infertility. Neither treatment has been evaluated in comparison with expectant management. IUI with superovulation is the more commonly used intervention. A single randomised trial showed that pregnancy rates in women treated by IUI alone were comparable to those in women treated by IUI with superovulation or IVF. A much larger multi-centre American trial found IUI with superovulation to be more effective than IUI alone in terms of live birth rates (OR 1.7, 95% CI 1.2–2.6) but the risk of multiple pregnancy was appreciably higher. IUI alone thus offers the safer option, while IUI with superovulation may enhance success rates but at the cost of a much higher multiple pregnancy rate.

GAMETE INTRAFALLOPIAN TRANSFER

Where the pelvis is normal, it is possible to consider gamete intrafallopian transfer (GIFT). This technique obviates the need for a sophisticated embryology laboratory but requires a laparoscopy under general anaesthetic. Results from two randomised trials suggest that the outcome following IUI with superovulation may be comparable to that achieved by GIFT. A third trial, however, suggests that GIFT is more effective. Given the more invasive nature of GIFT, it seems reasonable to offer a limited number of IUI cycles before progressing to GIFT or IVF. IVF has been shown to be comparable to GIFT in terms of live birth rates (OR 2.57, 95% CI 0.93–7.08) and more effective than GIFT in terms of pregnancy rates (OR 2.14, 95% CI 1.08–4.2).[5] It is also less invasive and more likely to provide important diagnostic information regarding fertilisation. In centres capable of offering IVF, this, rather than GIFT, should be the treatment of choice.

IN VITRO FERTILISATION

Treatment of unexplained infertility that is prolonged or refractory to other forms of treatment is undertaken by IVF. IVF also has a diagnostic role in identifying any problems with fertilisation and can circumvent most of the potential barriers to conception. Despite its widespread use in unexplained infertility, evidence supporting the role of IVF is limited. The possibility of failed fertilisation has prompted some workers to consider ICSI to be the definitive treatment of unexplained infertility. Evidence from a single randomised trial has failed to demonstrate any advantage of ICSI over IVF in the absence of male factor infertility.

OTHER MEDICAL TREATMENTS

There is no evidence to support the use of bromocriptine or danazol in the treatment of unexplained infertility.

KEY POINTS
- There is little justification for investigations other than biochemical tests for ovulation, semen analysis and pelvic assessment by laparoscopy.
- Outcome of unexplained infertility depends on the duration of infertility, female age and parity. While treatment must be tailored to the individual couple, active intervention is not recommended unless the duration of infertility is more than 3 years or the female partner is more than 35 years of age.

- Effective treatments include superovulation with IUI and in vitro fertilisation. There may be a role for empirical clomifene, while the effectiveness of unstimulated IUI needs to be demonstrated in the context of randomised trials.

Summary

Unexplained infertility continues to present a diagnostic and therapeutic challenge. Advances in assisted reproduction have improved outcome for many couples and simplified our management of the condition but many questions still remain unanswered.

KEY POINTS

- Unexplained infertility is a diagnosis of exclusion in the presence of normal semen parameters, evidence of ovulation and tubal patency.
- The main factors affecting outcome are duration of infertility, female age and parity.
- Expectant treatment is recommended unless the duration of infertility is more than 3 years or the female partner is more than 35 years of age.
- Effective treatments include superovulation with intrauterine insemination and in vitro fertilisation. The role of empirical clomifene is debatable.

References

1. National Collaborating Centre for Women's and Children's Health. *Fertility: Assessment and Treatment for People with Fertility Problems*. London: RCOG Press; 2004.
2. Collins JA, Rowe TC. Age of the female partner is a prognostic factor in prolonged unexplained infertility. *Fertil Steril* 1989;52:15–20.
3. Hughes E, Collins J, Vanderkove P. Clomiphene citrate vs placebo or no treatment in unexplained infertility. *Cochrane Database Syst Rev* 1998;(2).
4. Hughes EG. The effectiveness of ovulation induction and intrauterine insemination in the treatment of unexplained infertility: a meta-analysis. *Hum Reprod* 1997;12:1865–72.
5. Pandian Z, Bhattacharya S, Nicolau D, Vale L, Templeton A. In vitro fertilisation for unexplained subfertility. The effectiveness of in vitro fertilisation in unexplained infertility: a systematic review. *Hum Reprod* 2003;18:2001–7.

8 Assisted conception techniques

Introduction

Fifty percent of all couples with fertility problems will either conceive spontaneously or with the help of conventional treatment. In the remaining 50%, assisted reproduction techniques involving manipulation of the gametes (sperm or egg) may provide the final option.

This chapter focuses on the different techniques for assisted conception and the evidence supporting their use in everyday practice. The procedures, their technical basis, indications and results are summarised in Table 8.1.

Factors affecting the outcome of assisted reproduction treatment

AGE OF THE WOMAN

A woman's age is probably the most significant single predictor of live birth (Table 8.2). The optimal age range for treatment is 23–39 years, with the highest live birth rates being in the age group 25–30 years.

NUMBER OF PREVIOUS TREATMENT CYCLES

The chances of a live birth following IVF treatment are consistent for the first three cycles but effectiveness after three cycles becomes less certain.

PAST REPRODUCTIVE HISTORY

Women who have achieved a previous pregnancy, and particularly those with a previous live birth, have a significantly higher live birth rate compared with those who have had no previous pregnancies.

DURATION OF INFERTILITY

The duration of infertility is also a major factor in determining the likelihood of a spontaneous pregnancy. There is a significant decrease in

Table 8.1   Techniques used in assisted reproduction and outcomes

Technique	Principle	Major indications	Outcome (%)
IUI	Use of prepared partner's semen for insemination in a natural cycle or following ovulation induction	Unexplained infertility Mild male factor infertility	11[a]
IVF	Oocyte retrieval under ultrasound guidance. Insemination, embryo culture and transcervical replacement of embryos	Tubal disease Intractable pathology Failed primary treatment	24[b]
ICSI	IVF in which a single sperm is injected into the cytoplasm to allow fertilisation	Severe oligozoospermia in the male Failed fertilisation with IVF	26[b]
Donor insemination	Use of prepared donor semen for insemination	Azoospermia Infectious disease in the male partner Prevent transmission of genetic conditions	11[b]
Oocyte donation	Donor oocyte retrieval under ultrasound guidance and transcervical replacement of embryos into the recipient's endometrial cavity	Absent or non-functioning ovaries Prevent transmission of genetic conditions Repeated poor response with IVF treatment	25–28[b]

[a] pregnancy rate; [b] live birth rate

Table 8.2   Chances of a live birth following an IVF cycle

Age (years)	Live birth (%)
23–35	> 20
36–38	15
39	10
≥ 40	6

age-adjusted live birth rates with increasing duration of infertility between 1 and 12 years. Couples with a 12-year duration of infertility are half as likely to achieve a live birth compared with those with less than 3 years of infertility.

OVARIAN RESERVE

Assessment of ovarian reserve, which is a function of the total number of primordial follicles within the ovaries, has been used as a method of predicting the likelihood of a successful response to ovarian stimulation in the context of assisted reproduction treatment.

Several tests have been used to assess ovarian reserve. The sensitivity and specificity of most of these remains low and ovarian response during an assisted reproduction treatment cycle may well be the best predictor of reproductive outcome. Common tests include early follicular (day 3) serum FSH levels and the clomifene citrate challenge test. Antral follicular count and ovarian volume assessed using ultrasound scan have also been reported to be useful. Serum inhibin B and anti-müllerian hormone (AMH) levels are other tests which have also been considered as indirect measures of ovarian reserve. Currently available evidence suggests that existing tests of ovarian reserve have limited predictive value and hence routine use of these tests is not recommended.

SURGERY FOR HYDROSALPINGES BEFORE IVF TREATMENT

Hydrosalpinges have been shown to be associated with poor implantation, early pregnancy loss and lower live birth rates. This could be secondary to the toxic effect of the inflammatory fluid within the hydrosalpinx and possible alterations in endometrial receptivity. A systematic review of three randomised trials showed that surgical removal of the fallopian tube (salpingectomy), prior to IVF treatment, significantly increased live birth rates. The effect of draining hydrosalpinges or performing salpingostomy, on treatment outcome needs further evaluation.

IUI (with or without ovulation induction)

IUI involves timed introduction of washed motile sperm into the uterine cavity. Prior sperm preparation results in the removal of prostaglandins, bacteria and immunocompetent cells, thus reducing the risk of cramping and infection. Sperm preparation also increases the number of highly motile spermatozoa and removes dead or moribund spermatozoa and leukocytes that generate free oxygen radicals, which reduce the functional capacity of the spermatozoa. Ovarian stimulation by means of gonadotrophins or anti-estrogens to induce multiple ovulation has also been used in combination with IUI and, although more successful in achieving live birth, this is associated with an increased risk of multiple pregnancy. Pituitary downregulation is not employed and the ovarian response is monitored by serial ultrasound examinations and serum estrogen levels.

In unstimulated IUI, urine or serum LH levels are monitored in order to detect an LH surge, which determines the timing of insemination. Where superovulation is undertaken, ultrasound monitoring is generally commenced from days 10–12 of the cycle in order to assess the development of ovarian follicles. The aim is to achieve at least one follicle (no more than three) greater than 16 mm in diameter. When the leading follicle is 17 mm, a single dose of hCG is administered in order to induce the final steps of oocyte maturation and trigger ovulation. Insemination is carried out 24–48 hours later. In the presence of four or more follicles above 14 mm, cycle cancellation should be considered in view of a substantial risk of multiple pregnancy. Concurrent barrier contraception should also be recommended. Ovulation induction in anovulatory women is described in more detail in Chapter 4.

Indications for IUI (with or without ovulation induction) include:

- unexplained infertility
- mild male-factor infertility

- coital or ejaculatory disorders
- donor insemination.

KEY POINTS
- Unstimulated IUI is a relatively less invasive technique and should be considered in preference to stimulated IUI, especially in cases of mild male factor infertility.
- Ovarian stimulation is associated with an increased risk of multiple pregnancy.
- If four or more follicles develop, couples should be advised to cancel the treatment cycle.

In vitro fertilisation

IVF is a method of assisted reproduction where sperm and oocytes are mixed to allow fertilisation to occur in vitro. The resulting embryos are subsequently transferred within the cavity of the uterus. The technique, first developed by Edwards and Steptoe, was used to overcome tubal disease and has probably been one of the most significant developments in the management of infertility. Since the birth of the first 'test tube baby', Louise Brown, in 1978, the technique has been further refined and indications for its use have expanded to cover all cases of unresolved infertility irrespective of cause.

OVARIAN STIMULATION

Ovarian stimulation is used to promote the development of a relatively synchronous cohort of follicles. The aim is to achieve a satisfactory yield of mature oocytes without risking ovarian hyperstimulation.

Ovarian stimulation has traditionally been achieved using hMG or purified urinary FSH. More recently, recombinant gonadotrophins (r-FSH and r-LH) have become available. A meta-analysis of randomised controlled trials comparing r-FSH with the less expensive urinary-derived product showed both to be equally effective in achieving a live birth following IVF. Ovulation induction is described in more detail in Chapter 4.

Pituitary downregulation (desensitisation) using GnRH analogues is often employed prior to and during ovarian stimulation to suppress endogenous LH and minimise the risk of a premature LH surge. It has been shown to increase the clinical pregnancy rates in the context of IVF, as it reduces the risk of cycle cancellation. It also has practical advantages in terms of greater flexibility in timing and scheduling treatment cycles.

GnRH analogues have been used in long, short and ultra-short protocols. In the long protocol, they are started either in the early follicular or in the mid-luteal phase and given for 14–21 days, after which gonadotrophins are commenced. In the short protocol, GnRH analogues are administered for 10–14 days, usually commencing at the beginning of the stimulation cycle, while in the ultra-short protocol they are used for about 3 days at the beginning of the stimulation cycle. Both short and ultra-short protocols take advantage of the increased secretion of gonadotrophins resulting from the initial direct stimulation of the pituitary gland before achieving down-regulation. A systematic review of 26 randomised controlled trials (RCTs) found increased clinical pregnancy rates with the long compared with the short and ultra-short protocols. At present the long protocol is the one most commonly used in standard clinical practice.

GnRH antagonists produce direct and immediate pituitary suppression. Two systematic reviews (including six RCTs) showed that the use of GnRH antagonist resulted in reduced clinical pregnancy rates when compared to the long GnRH analogue protocol. There was no significant difference in the multiple pregnancy rate, miscarriage rate, cycle cancellation rate or the incidence of severe OHSS. Patient satisfaction, however, was not considered in these reviews. Many women could find these agents more user friendly, as they shorten the treatment cycle and avoid the estrogen withdrawal effects associated with GnRH analogues. The National Institute for Health and Clinical Excellence (NICE) guideline for the management of infertility recommends that, at present, the use of GnRH antagonists should only be within a research context.[1]

Monitoring ovarian response is essential to ensure safe practice, to reduce the risk of OHSS and to optimise the timing of oocyte retrieval. Evidence from two RCTs suggests that monitoring estrogen levels during ovulation induction does not give additional information with regard to pregnancy rates or the incidence of OHSS when compared with ultra-sound monitoring alone.

In terms of triggering ovulation, recombinant hCG has been shown to be comparable to urinary hCG in terms of pregnancy rates and incidence of OHSS.

OOCYTE RETRIEVAL

Oocyte retrieval is carried out using transvaginal ultrasound-guided needle aspiration. This is usually performed under light sedation and analgesia. Combinations of benzodiazepines and opiates are administered either intravenously or intramuscularly. A survey of current practice in the UK reported that 84% of IVF clinics used intravenous sedation while 16% used general anaesthesia for transvaginal ultrasound-guided oocyte retrieval. General anaesthetics could traverse into the follicular fluid and might be detrimental to the cleavage of the embryos and pregnancy rates. Conscious sedation allows the patient to remain awake and to be accompanied by her partner. Conscious sedation also requires less specialised equipment, avoids possible complications associated with general anaesthetic and is usually well tolerated by women, although there is a theoretical risk of the agents used contaminating the follicular fluid. The NICE guideline for the management of infertility recommends that women undergoing transvaginal oocyte retrieval should be offered conscious sedation as a safe and acceptable method of providing analgesia.[1]

Oocyte recovery usually takes 15–30 minutes and is carried out using a single or double lumen needle, attached to an electronic pump, which enables rapid aspiration of the follicles. The double lumen needles also allow 'flushing' of the follicles in situations where the oocytes are not obtained from the initial aspirate. A total of three RCTs compared a policy of routinely flushing the follicles with no flushing and showed no difference in the number of oocytes retrieved or in pregnancy rates. The use of follicle flushing in women with fewer than three follicles has not been evaluated but flushing may be useful for ensuring that the oocyte yield is maximised. Possible complications of oocyte retrieval include vascular and visceral injury (0.2%), pelvic infection (0.4%) and adnexal torsion (0.1%).

INSEMINATION

After oocyte retrieval, freshly ejaculated seminal fluid is prepared to concentrate motile spermatozoa in a fraction that is free of seminal plasma and debris. Insemination is usually performed 1–6 hours after oocyte retrieval with 50 000–200 000 motile spermatozoa for each oocyte. Following an incubation period of 16–18 hours in suitable culture media, oocytes are examined to ensure that normal fertilisation, as defined by the presence of two pronuclei, has occurred. Abnormal fertilisation occurs in 5% of fertilised oocytes and is generally attributed to polyspermy or non-extrusion of the second polar body. Such oocytes are not suitable for transfer. Suitable embryos are kept in culture within the incubator at 37°C and in a humid atmosphere containing 5% CO_2 until they are either transferred into the uterine cavity or cryopreserved.

MICRO-ASSISTED FERTILISATION

ICSI implies using micromanipulation to aid fertilisation and involves the direct injection of a single sperm through the outer membrane of the oocyte into the cytoplasm (Figure 8.1). Since the birth of the first child

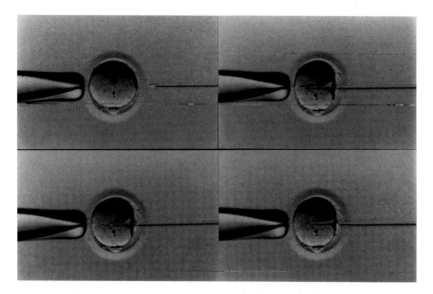

Figure 8.1 Injection of a single spermatozoa into an oocyte

resulting from ICSI treatment in 1993, this treatment has revolutionised the management of couples suffering from severe male-factor infertility.

The main indications for ICSI include very poor semen quality, following surgical sperm extraction and previous failed fertilisation in an IVF cycle. There is no difference between IVF and ICSI in terms of pregnancy rates when used in couples with non-male factor subfertility.

Micromanipulation of the embryo in the form of 'assisted hatching' has been proposed as a method to disrupt the zona pellucida to facilitate and enhance implantation and pregnancy rates. A systematic review of 23 RCTs showed no increase in the live birth rate with assisted hatching. There was an overall increase in clinical pregnancy rates, although these results should be interpreted with caution because of the poor methodological quality of the studies included in the review. There is thus insufficient evidence to support the routine use of assisted hatching.

Safety concerns have been expressed regarding the use of micromanipulation techniques, especially ICSI, in view of the limited knowledge about the natural selection of the spermatozoa for fertilisation. Some studies have shown a slightly higher relative risk of congenital abnormalities, including chromosomal anomalies in children conceived through IVF and ICSI, although the absolute risks remain low. Some of these findings may reflect transmission of existing chromosomal defects in the parents. Further long-term follow up studies are needed.

EMBRYO TRANSFER

In IVF cycles, embryo transfer is usually performed 48 hours following the oocyte collection (four-cell stage). A systematic review of trials comparing a 48-hour versus 72-hour transfer policy concluded that there is insufficient evidence to show a clear benefit of one over the other.

Studies have assessed prolonged in vitro culture to the blastocyst stage (day 5–6) prior to replacing the embryos. The rationale for blastocyst culture is to improve the synchronicity of uterine and embryonic development and provide a mechanism for self-selection of viable embryos. Transfer on days 5–6 shows no clear evidence of benefit in terms of live birth rate per cycle started but may result in a lower number of women proceeding to an embryo transfer.

No randomised trials have compared two- versus three-embryo transfer. A review of the Human Fertilisation and Embryology Authority (HFEA) data (1991–1995), however, showed that, when more than two eggs were fertilised, the transfer of three embryos did not increase the chances of a live birth (over the transfer of two embryos) but significantly increased the risk of both twin and triplet births. Subsequently, the HFEA sixth Code of Practice[2] stated that no more than two embryos should be transferred in any one treatment cycle in women aged less than 40 years, while those aged 40 years or over may receive up to a maximum of three embryos.

A systematic review of four trials showed that in women under 36 years of age, transferring one fresh embryo and then, if needed, one frozen and thawed embryo reduces the rate of multiple births while achieving live birth rates not substantially lower than those with a double-embryo transfer. Further research is needed to evaluate this.

A meta-analysis of RCTs that assessed the use of ultrasound guided embryo transfer showed a significant increase in pregnancy rates with routine ultrasound guided embryo transfer. Replacement of embryos into a uterine cavity with an endometrium of less than 5 mm thickness is unlikely to result in a pregnancy and is therefore not recommended.

LUTEAL PHASE SUPPORT

The aspiration of the granulosa cells that surround the oocytes and the use of GnRH analogues for pituitary downregulation can interfere with the production of progesterone during the luteal phase, which is necessary for successful implantation of the embryo. Hormonal supplementation during the luteal phase using either progesterone or hCG (which stimulates progesterone production) improves implantation and increases pregnancy rates. The routine use of hCG, however, is not recommended, as it does not provide better results compared with progesterone and is associated with a greater risk of OHSS.

SUCCESS RATES OF TREATMENT

Success rates for IVF have risen significantly during the course of the last 10 years and have recently reached 28.8% live birth rate/embryo transfer for women under the age of 38 years and 24.3% for all ages. Success rates for ICSI have been similar to those reported for IVF with 28.7% live birth rate per embryo transfer for women under the age of 38 years and 25.7% for all ages.[1]

CRYOPRESERVATION OF EMBRYOS AND GAMETES

Embryo cryopreservation is now firmly established as a routine component of IVF. Cryopreservation allows supernumerary embryos resulting from the initial oocyte retrieval procedure to be stored and replaced in subsequent attempts. This increases the number of potential embryo replacement cycles while reducing the risks of ovarian stimulation and surgical oocyte retrieval. Embryos are usually frozen at pronuclear or early cleavage stage. Embryos are stored in liquid nitrogen at −196°C and 70% of embryos are expected to survive after thawing. The most important factor affecting post-thaw survival is embryo quality. Thawed embryos are transferred 2–3 days after a luteal surge in carefully monitored natural cycles. Alternatively, embryos can be replaced in artificial cycles in which downregulation using GnRH analogues is followed by stimulation of the endometrium using sequential HRT (estradiol followed by estradiol and progesterone). While the superiority of either method has yet to be proven conclusively, there is a reported age-related decline in pregnancy rates with natural replacement cycles that is not evident in hormonally stimulated cycles. Live birth rates following frozen embryo transfer are generally lower than those for fresh treatment cycles, with overall figures reported to be about 11.5%. Several factors, including the transfer of the 'better quality' embryos at the fresh cycles, might contribute to this difference. The HFEA permits embryo storage for up to 10 years, although there is no evidence that storage beyond this period affects embryo quality or congenital malformation rates or perinatal outcome.

Semen cryopreservation is considered in men with malignancies facing chemotherapy or radiotherapy that can affect fertility. This provides an opportunity to preserve fertility and for the sperm to be used for assisted fertilisation at a later date. Evidence from animal research shows no decline in sperm viability with time and hence would suggest no biological time limit to cryopreservation.

Cryopreservation of oocytes has a limited success rate, although live births have been reported following ICSI used for fertilisation of cryopreserved oocytes. Cryopreservation of ovarian tissue followed by autografting or in vitro culture has been suggested and may be a valuable option in conserving fertility. This, however, is still at an early stage of development and more research is needed to explore this area.

KEY POINTS
- The advent of ICSI treatment has revolutionised the management of couples suffering from male-factor infertility.
- No more than two embryos should be transferred in any one treatment cycle.
- Further research is awaited on the role of a single embryo transfer policy.

Gamete intrafallopian transfer

GIFT is a procedure where gametes (oocyte and sperm) are transferred laparoscopically into the fallopian tube at the time of oocyte collection. Fertilisation takes place, in vivo, within the fallopian tube. GIFT has been most commonly used in the management of couples with unexplained or mild male factor infertility.

Controlled ovarian stimulation in GIFT is the same as in IVF and the procedure requires women with healthy and patent fallopian tubes. Drawbacks associated with GIFT include the need for general anaesthesia and laparoscopy and the inability to confirm fertilisation.

Zygote intrafallopian transfer

Zygote intrafallopian transfer (ZIFT) is a technique that has been developed alongside IVF and involves the laparoscopic transfer of embryos into the fallopian tubes after fertilisation in vitro. There is insufficient evidence, at present, to recommend the use of GIFT or ZIFT in preference to IVF.

Donor insemination

The introduction of ICSI allowed many couples with severe male factor infertility, who would have otherwise resorted to donor insemination, to have their own genetic children. The main indications for treatment by donor insemination include:

- azoospermia (obstructive or non obstructive, see Chapter 3)
- infectious disease in the male partner (such as HIV or hepatitis)
- following chemotherapy or radiotherapy
- to prevent the transmission of a genetic disorder to the offspring
- severe rhesus isoimmunisation with a homozygous rhesus-positive male partner.

Donor recruitment is performed in accordance with the British Andrology Society Consensus Guidelines.[3] The selection and screening of sperm donors allows the protection of the offspring resulting from the treatment of heritable genetic disorders and the recipient women from infection. The HFEA Code of Practice[2] sets an upper age limit of 45 years for sperm donors. In accordance with the British Andrology Society Consensus Guidelines, donors in the UK are offered the following screening tests:

- karyotyping
- screening for autosomal recessive disorders (such as cystic fibrosis, beta thalassaemia, sickle cell disease and Tay Sachs disease)
- screening for rhesus antigens
- *Chlamydia trachomatis*
- HIV
- hepatitis B and C
- syphilis
- cytomegalovirus (CMV).

The British Andrology Society Consensus Guidelines recommend a mandatory quarantine period for donor sperm of 6 months prior to its use to minimise the risk of sexually transmitted viral infections.[3]

All couples that undergo donor insemination should be offered independent counselling to explain the implications of treatment, both for themselves and for potential resulting children. They need to understand how donors are selected and screened and the limitations of accurate matching. The counsellor should also describe the law with respect to the legal position of the child and the parents and the rules governing confidentiality and anonymity.

Women receiving donor insemination should be offered tests to confirm their ovulation and those with a history suggestive of tubal damage should be offered tubal assessment before treatment.

The NICE guidelines for the management of infertility recommend that women with no risk factors for tubal disease should be offered tubal assessment after three unsuccessful treatment cycles. Ovarian stimulation is only indicated for anovulatory cycles, while for those with ovulatory cycles, insemination is timed to coincide with ovulation. This is usually determined by daily monitoring of serum LH levels or by urinary LH detection kit. The live birth rates following donor insemination, for each cycle started, are 12% for women below 38 years of age and 11% for all ages. Live birth rates following donor insemination decrease with increasing woman's age and women over 40 years old have only a 3–4% chance of success following each donor insemination treatment cycle.

KEY POINTS
- Sperm is cryopreserved for a 6-month quarantine period to allow for donor screening tests to be completed and minimise the risk of sexually transmitted infections.
- All couples wishing to undergo donor insemination should receive independent counselling.
- Ovarian stimulation is only indicated for anovulatory cycles.

Ovum donation

The main indications for using donor oocytes include the following:
- premature ovarian failure (primary or secondary)
- bilateral oophorectomy
- irreversible gonadal damage following certain regimens of chemotherapy or radiotherapy
- gonadal dysgenesis associated with Turner syndrome or other chromosomal disorders
- high risk of transmitting a genetic disorder to the offspring
- certain cases of repeated IVF failure, including markedly diminished ovarian reserve, poor quality oocytes and unexplained failure of fertilisation.

Success rates are primarily dependent on the age of the donor. It is, therefore, recommended that egg donors should be no older than 35 years at the time of donation, as success rates for assisted conception significantly decrease beyond that. However, with the increasing age of the recipient, there is also a tendency to a decline in success rates, possibly due to endometrial ageing. Success rates for IVF using donated eggs have been reported to be similar in women with and without primary ovarian failure.

Before donation is undertaken, oocyte donors should be screened for infectious and genetic diseases in accordance with the guidance issued by the HFEA (see screening for donor insemination).

Donors and recipients should be offered independent counselling regarding the physical and psychological implications of treatment for themselves and their genetic children. Careful counselling regarding the potential risks of ovarian stimulation and the oocyte retrieval procedure should also be undertaken.

Donors undergo ovarian stimulation as in IVF cycles. The collected oocytes are inseminated with the recipient's partner's sperm and the resulting embryos are transferred into the recipient's uterus. It is usually necessary to provide the recipient with HRT, using sequential oral doses of estrogens followed by progestogens to mimic the natural cyclical hormonal pattern. Recipients who have a spontaneous menstrual cycle require pituitary desensitisation before commencing the HRT regimen, while women with ovarian failure who are amenorrhoeic do not.

KEY POINTS
- Independent counselling is required for both the recipient couple and the donor.
- Donors undergo ovarian stimulation, as in IVF cycles.

DONOR ANONYMITY

Under existing regulations in the UK, people donating sperm, eggs or embryos have remained anonymous. Following a Department of Health announcement in January 2004, a change in the law means that children born as a result of sperm, eggs or embryos donated after April 2005 can access the identity of their donor when they reach the age of 18 years. The new regulations surrounding information on donors are retrospective so anybody donating before April 2005 will remain anonymous.

Many people believe that children born from donated sperm, eggs or embryos should be able to have access to information about their genetic origins, as this may have an important role in the formation of their personal identity. Furthermore, concealment of such information could have a detrimental effect on the individual's familial and social relationships, particularly if that information is later discovered in an unplanned manner. It is acknowledged that ending donor anonymity does involve some risk to the future availability of donors, although research from other countries where anonymity had been removed is reassuring in this respect. In 1985, Sweden changed its laws to allow all donor insemination offspring the right to obtain identifying information about the donor. This resulted in an initial reduction in donors although subsequently the number of donors coming forward returned to its original levels.

Surrogacy

Surrogacy in the UK is regulated under the Surrogacy Arrangements Act 1985 and is carried out within premises licensed by the HFEA. Indications for surrogacy include surgical removal or congenital absence of the uterus and medical conditions as severe cardiac disease or liver disease.

By law, the carrying mother is the legal mother (that is, the surrogate mother in a surrogacy arrangement). This has a number of implications. In order for the intended parents to become the legal parents of the child, they must either apply to adopt the child or apply for a parental order. This would also apply if they were the genetic parents of the child (their sperm and eggs were used).

Definitions

Complete surrogacy: Sperm from the partner of the infertile woman is used to inseminate the surrogate mother, who will carry the pregnancy and give the resulting child over to the couple. The couple then adopts the child.

Partial surrogacy: The woman has intact ovaries but is unable to gestate due to an absent or severely malformed uterus. The couple can create an embryo in vitro, then have it transferred to the uterus of the surrogate host.

The ethical aspects of surrogacy are considerable and it is essential that the surrogate host and her partner as well as the couple receive independent counselling before embarking upon treatment.

Welfare of the child

The HFEA Act states that, before assisted conception treatment is offered, account must be taken for the welfare of any child that may be born as a result of the treatment. It would be expected that medical and physical risks as well as psychological and social factors that could impact on the welfare of the child are considered in the process. This also covers issues related to growing up in a particular family structure, such as single parent families, same sex parents, older parents, those in which one or both parents are not genetically related to their children or those created through surrogacy arrangements.

Human Fertilisation and Embryology Authority

The regulation of infertility treatment in the UK is undertaken by the HFEA, which was established following the Human Fertilisation and Embryology Act 1990. The first statutory body of its type in the world, the HFEA's creation reflected public and professional concern about the implications that new techniques for assisted reproduction might have on the perception of human life and family relationships.

The HFEA's principle task is to regulate, by means of a system of licensing, audit and inspection, any treatment or research that involves the creation, keeping and use of human embryos outside the body. The HFEA also regulates the storage or donation of gametes (sperm and eggs) and embryos.

Summary

The development of IVF has had a major impact on the provision of fertility treatment. Since its introduction it has found wide application in the management of couples with ovulatory disorders, endometriosis, unexplained infertility and tubal factor infertility. The introduction of micro-assisted fertilisation in the form of ICSI has re-shaped the management of couples with severe male factor infertility. It has allowed many men to parent their own genetic children where, in the past, their only option would have been to resort to donor sperm.

A two-embryo transfer is favoured over a three-embryo transfer. This significantly reduces the risk of triplet pregnancy without compromising live birth rates and clinics throughout the UK have now applied this policy. Early research on single embryo transfer is promising and more research would be eagerly awaited to evaluate the role of such a policy in standard practice. This could have significant implications in reducing the risk of multiple pregnancy and subsequently a reduction in neonatal as well as maternal morbidity.

Current research is largely reassuring on the health and wellbeing of children born as a result of assisted reproduction. The rational development and deployment of IVF and the techniques of micro-assisted fertilisation holds at least the promise of a solution for many couples. For clinicians, the challenge is to deploy these new techniques safely and effectively.

References

1. National Collaborating Centre for Women's and Children's Health. *Fertility: Assessment and Treatment for People with Fertility Problems.* London: RCOG Press; 2004.
2. Human Fertilisation and Embryology Authority. *Code of Practice.* 6th ed. London: The Stationery Office; 2003.
3. British Andrology Society. Consensus guidelines for the screening of semen donors for donor insemination. *Hum Reprod* 1999;1:1823–6.

Further reading

Templeton A, Cooke I, O'Brien PMS, editors. *Evidence-based Fertility Treatment.* London: RCOG Press; 1998.

Index

C

cabergoline 62
cancer
  risk of 8, 59
  treatment 29
causes of infertility 3–4
cervical mucus, postcoital test 19
chemicals, toxic 29
chemotherapy 29
child, welfare of 111–12
Chlamydia trachomatis infections
  prevention 5, 77
  screening 18, 19, 77
  tubal infertility 3, 66–7
  unexplained infertility 91
chromosomal abnormalities 28–9, 33, 44–5
cimetidine 29
clinics, infertility 9, 20
clomifene 51–2
  adverse effects 8, 52, 58
  challenge test 99
  and dexamethasone 53
  effectiveness 52
  and hCG 53
  in male factor infertility 40
  mechanism of action 51
  in ovulatory dysfunction 49, 50, 51
  treatment regimes 51–2
  in unexplained infertility 93–4
cocaine 34
coital dysfunction 26–7
colchicine 29
congenital abnormalities
  genital tract 68
  IVF– and ICSI-conceived children 104
congenital bilateral absence of vas
    deferens (CBAVD) 33
consultation, infertility 12–13
context of care 9–10
cost effectiveness, infertility treatments 6
counselling 7
  for donor insemination 108
  general advice 17, 18
  for oocyte donation 110
  in ovulatory dysfunction 48
  in psychosexual dysfunction 37
  in tubal factor infertility 71
couple, infertile
  context of care 9
  general advice 17, 18

initial assessment 11–21
cryopreservation
  gametes and embryos 106–7
  sperm 33, 42, 106
cystic fibrosis 28, 33
cytokines, in endometriosis 83
cytotoxic drugs 29

D

danazol 95
dehydroepiandrosterone sulphate
    (DHEA-S) 46
dexamethasone, and clomifene 53
diabetes, type 2 48
diagnostic categories, infertility 4
dibromochloropropane (DBCP) 29
diet, in ovulation disorders 60
DNA analysis 33
donor insemination (DI) 41, 98, 107–9
donors, anonymity 110–11
dopamine agonists 36, 62
doxycycline 68
drugs, causing male infertility 29
duration of infertility 6
  outcome of assisted conception and
    97–9
  in unexplained infertility 92, 93

E

E_2 (estradiol), serum 54, 57
ectopic pregnancy 71, 77
eggs *see* oocytes
ejaculation, retrograde 26, 27
  treatment 37
ejaculatory duct obstruction 28
ejaculatory failure 26
ejaculatory problems 26
  management 37–8
electroejaculation 37
embryos
  assisted hatching 104
  cryopreservation 106–7
  culture 103, 105
  donors 110–11
  impaired implantation 82
  number transferred 8, 105, 112
  transfer 105
emotional consequences, infertility 7
empirical treatment
  male factor infertility 39–41
  unexplained infertility 93–4

ultrasound scans 46–8
ovulation
    investigations 16, 44
    suppression, in endometriosis 84
ovulation induction 49, 50–5
    for donor insemination 108–9
    GnRH agonists 60–1
    for IUI 100
    for IVF 101–2
    in male factor infertility 41
    for oocyte donation 110
    in unexplained infertility 93–4
    unwanted effects 7–8, 56–9
ovulatory dysfunction 4, 43–64
    classification 43–4, 45
    diagnosis 44–8
    in endometriosis 81
    treatment 48–61
ovum donation 109–11
oxedrine 37

P

paracentesis, in ovarian hyperstimulation
    syndrome 58
PCOS *see* polycystic ovarian syndrome
pelvic inflammatory disease (PID) 65–7
    pathology 68
    prevention 77
pelvic investigations 17–19
pelvic surgery 68, 77
peritoneal environment, in endometriosis
    82–3
phenylpropanolamine hydrochloride 37
phosphodiesterase inhibitors, type 5 38
pioglitazone 50
pituitary disorders
    female infertility 44, 60–3
    male infertility 25–6
pituitary tumours 27, 44
    investigations 32
    treatment 61–3
polycystic ovarian syndrome (PCOS) 44
    diagnosis 45, 46–8
    laparoscopic ovarian drilling 55
    treatment 49–55
polycystic ovaries 46
postcoital test (PCT) 19, 20, 33, 92
pregnancy loss, subclinical 90
prevalence of infertility 2
prevention of infertility 5
primary care 9

initial assessment 11–12
    see also general practitioner
primary infertility 1, 4
progesterone
    in endometriosis 81–2
    luteal phase support in IVF 105–6
    serum 16, 44
prolactin
    elevated levels *see* hyperprolactinaemia
    serum 16, 31–2, 45
prostatovesiculitis 27–8
protocols, clinical 11, 20
psychological factors, in unexplained
    infertility 91
psychosexual dysfunction 26, 37
psychotherapy, in ovulation disorders 60
pyosalpinx 69

Q

quinogalide 62

R

radiotherapy 29
reproductive health, definition 1
reproductive history, past 97
rosiglitazone 50
rubella immune status 15

S

salpingectomy, in hydrosalpinx 75, 99
salpingography, selective, with tubal
    cannulation 71–3
salpingo-oophoritis 69
scrotum
    temperature 17, 18, 34
    ultrasound scan 32
secondary care 9
secondary infertility 1, 4, 6
sedation, for oocyte retrieval 102–3
semen
    analysis 13–15, 31
    cryopreservation 33, 42, 106
    microbiological assessment 32
    normal values 16
sex hormone-binding globulin (SHBG) 16
sexual dysfunction 19, 20, 26–7
    investigations 31–2
    management 37–8
sexually transmitted diseases (STD) 27–8,
    66–7
Sheehan syndrome 44

venography, retrograde 32
Viagra (sildenafil) 38
vitamin C 40
vitamin E 40

W

weight
    gain 45, 60
    loss 46, 49–50
welfare of child 111–12
white blood cells, in semen 32

World Health Organization (WHO)
    classification of ovulatory dysfunction 45
    semen analysis values 16
    survey on male factor infertility 23, 24

Y

Y chromosome microdeletions 33

Z

zygote intrafallopian transfer (ZIFT) 107